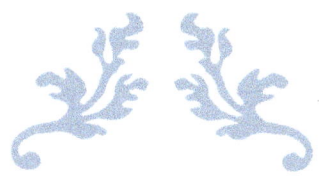

PALEO DIET COOKBOOK
FOR BEGINNERS

100 fast and easy recipes to start eating healthy, boost metabolism
and lose weight quickly

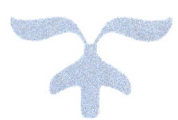

JESSICA COLLINS

this book has been derived from various sources. Please consult a licensed professional before attempting any techniques outlined in this book.

By reading this document, the reader agrees that under no circumstances is the author responsible for any losses, direct or indirect, which are incurred as a result of the use of information contained within this document, including, but not limited to, errors, omissions, or inaccuracies.

Table of Contents

INTRODUCTION

The paleo diet is eating that is concentrating on foods that our caveman ancestors would have eaten. It is a relatively simple diet, but it does require quite a bit of work. You need to eat unprocessed foods, limit your salt intake, eat healthy fats, and eat some fruit.

It allows you to avoid foods that have been associated with the disease. It helps reduce food cravings as it doesn't contain processed food full of sugar, fat, and carbs. It helps you to make better decisions as you can be more in tune with your body's needs. It is a low-carb, high protein diet, so it aids in weight loss and muscle gain. It is high in fat, so it suppresses hunger while providing energy for your body.

The paleo diet has several benefits for you. It is a very healthy diet that can help improve your body's overall health because you are not eating processed foods. Your diet will also help you look better and feel better as it removes junk food from your system.

Using the paleo diet cookbook can help you stick to the diet for the long term. All recipes are made with easy ingredients that focus on whole foods as opposed to processed products. As a bonus, all recipes are gluten-free! The paleo diet is appraised by many to be a healthy and balanced eating plan. This diet is based on the reliance that our body was meant to eat foods naturally. It primarily focuses on whole foods like fruits, vegetables, nuts, and seeds rather than processed foods to supply all of the necessary vitamins, minerals, and other nutrients to maintain and improve your health.

The paleo diet has been obtaining popularity over the last few years, especially among those interested in losing weight and enhance their overall health. Many people believe that this eating plan helps achieve both of those goals. The paleo diet cookbook is designed for beginners who are new to this eating plan.

The paleo diet encourages consuming whole foods with minimal processing or cooking. You can enjoy foods like meats, kinds of seafood, eggs, fruits, vegetables, and nuts without the addition of oils or other unhealthy additives. The paleo diet adopts high-fiber consumption and plenty of fruits and vegetables to help you stay healthy and fit. The paleo diet is a program that focuses on eating like it did in the Paleolithic Era. The paleo diet's mantra is that humans have an innate tendency to eat like our hunter-gatherer ancestors.

The paleo diet is constructed on the idea that modern man has become out-of-sync with his physiology. This out-of-sync can be attributed to the introduction of agriculture in the Neolithic era, which displaced our ancient hunter-gatherer ancestors. The theory goes that modern man is no longer fulfilling his physical requirements for food.

Many people of all ages have adopted this eating pattern out of a desire to lose weight and feel healthier and get a boost in their energy levels. Whether you want to drop a couple of pounds or you want a healthier lifestyle, paleo diet cookbooks can help you on your way. Throughout history, our ancient ancestors were hunters and gatherers. They spent their days searching for food and gathering around campfires to share stories and survival tips. They did not have access to modern conveniences such as farming or cooking, so they were highly selective about what they ate. Their food choices were built on what was available at the time, whether it was safe to eat or tasted good. This is why we see many similarities between paleo diet principles and eating habits among our ancient ancestors.

Today, we gather most of our days indoors and in front of computer screens. Taking care of business means having access to many different types of food during the day, but when you're Paleo, you are only allowed to eat foods that were available to our ancient ancestors. Due to this reason alone, many people believe that the Paleo Diet is an effective way to lose weight or gaining a healthy lifestyle. Many people who follow this diet have claimed that it helped relieve joint pain, balance blood sugar levels, lower cholesterol levels, and even help with allergies.

It's a diet that utilizes the foods that our ancestors ate and eliminates the foods they didn't. The paleo diet uses healthy grains, nuts, and meat along with vegetables. It also excludes dairy. The basic idea behind Paleo is to eat whole foods and avoid processed foods.

This is a guide for people that are looking for a dietary change that can benefit their health. It takes you step by step to follow the paleo diet, including how to choose paleo-friendly foods. We've included recipes for every meal, so you can easily find tasty dishes to fit this diet. We've even included tips on cooking the most popular recipes in the paleo cookbook so you can prepare your meals right at home. The recipes are available in print or for download as PDFs, which means that you'll be ready to go at a moment's notice!

If you're looking for a way to change up your dietary routine, this paleo cookbook has what you need! Stock up now and have a tastier way of eating soon!

BREAKFAST

1. Avocado Burger With Salmon

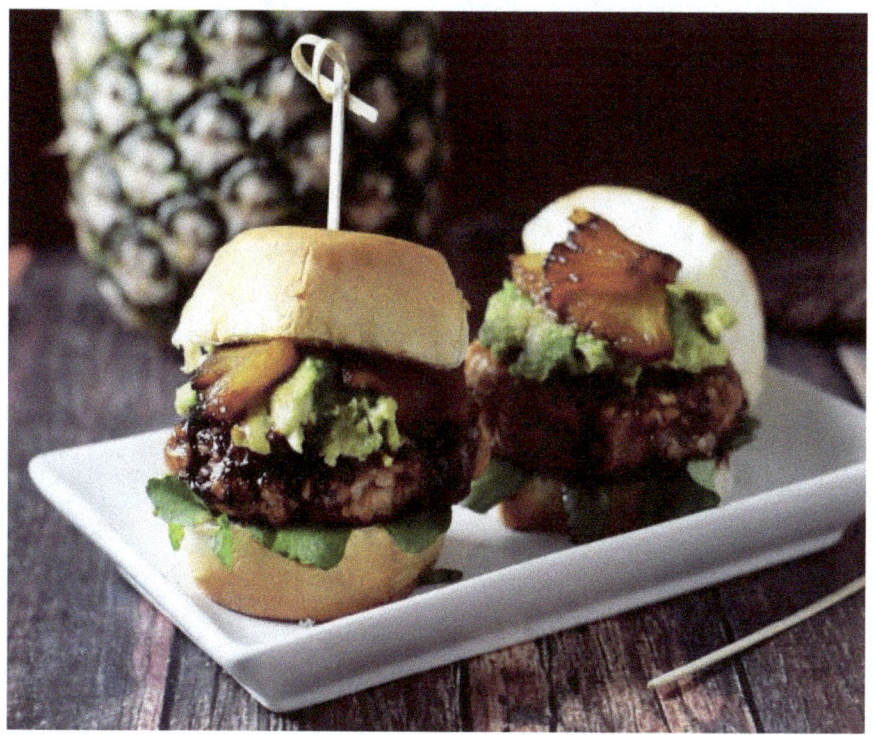

Preparation time: 10 minutes

Cooking Time: 20 minutes

Servings: 1

Ingredients:

- 1 Avocado

- 2 Slices Of Smoked Salmon

- Sesame Seeds

Directions:

1. Cut the avocado in half.

2. Peel it.

3. Remove the core.

4. Place the smoked salmon in between the two an avocado part.

5. Add some sesame seeds.

Nutrition:

Calories 60

Fat 2.3

Fiber 0.8

Carbs 5

Protein 5.6

2. Banana Mango Smoothie

Preparation time: 5 minutes

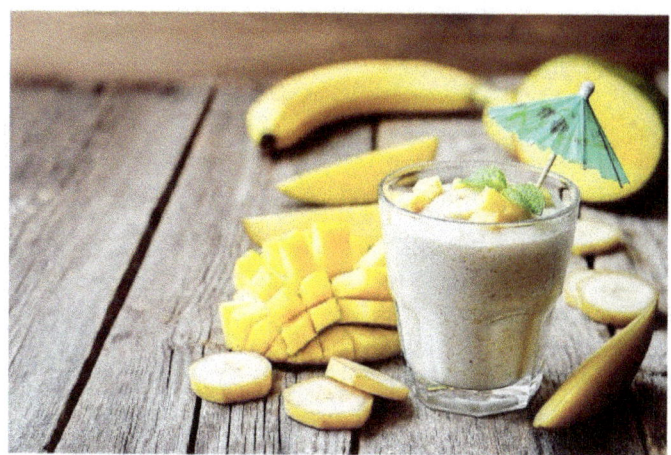

Cooking Time: 10 minutes

Servings: 1

Ingredients:

- 1 Banana

- 1 Mango

- 1 Cup Of Coconut Milk

Directions:

1. Peel the banana and slice it.

2. Peel the mango and cut it.

3. Use a mixer to whisk the fruits and milk together, keep some
   pieces of fruits for decoration.

4. Serve the smoothie in a glass and decorate it.

Nutrition:

Calories: 32

Fat: 5

Fiber: 2

Carbs: 11

Protein: 4

3. American Breakfast

Preparation time: 2 minutes

Cooking time: 5 minutes

Servings: 1

Ingredients:

- 2 Eggs

- 1/2 Cup Almond Milk

- 6 Slices Of Bacon

- Vegetable Oil

Directions:

1. Set the eggs in a bowl and whisk.

2. Add the milk

3. Preheat 2 pans over medium heat.

4. In one pan cook the bacon for about 5 minutes

5. In the other pan add some vegetable oil and scramble the eggs.

Nutrition:

Calories: 13

Fat: 4

Fiber: 5

Carbs: 23

Protein: 8

4. Chocolate Brownies

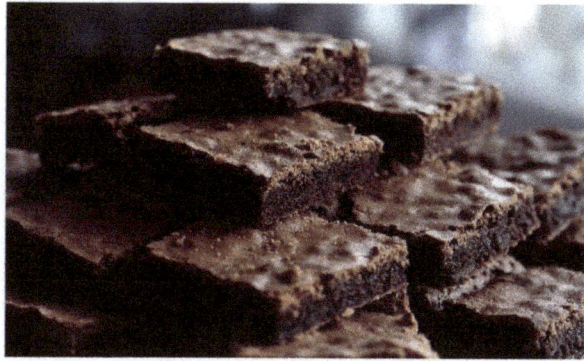

Preparation time: 10 minutes

Cooking time: 25 minutes

Servings: 3

Ingredients:

- 4 Eggs

- 1/2 Cup Cocoa Powder

- 2 Cups Of Almonds Okra

- 6 Tbsp. Of Honey

- 1 Tsp. Of Vanilla Powder

- Salt

- 1 Tsp. Of Baking Soda

- Coconut Oil

Directions:

1. In a bowl set the eggs and beat them with the honey.

2. Add the warm coconut oil and mix.

3. In another bowl mix the okra with the cocoa powder, the vanilla powder, the salt and baking soda.

4. Mix the two bowls ingredients together.

5. Pour the ingredients in a baking tin and cook in the oven for 25 minutes (340 F).

Nutrition:

Calories: 32

Fat: 5

Fiber: 2

Carbs: 11

Protein: 4

5. Almond Milk Homemade

Preparation time: 10 minutes

Cooking Time: 15 minutes

Servings: 1 bottle of almond milk

Ingredients

- 2 Cups Of Shelled Organic Almonds

- A Pinch Of Salt

- 4 Cups Of Still Water

- 1 Filter Bag FOR VEGETABLE MILK

Directions:

1. Put 4 cups of still water in a glass container, dip the almonds in the water and add a pinch of salt.

2. Let the almonds dip in the water for 12 hours. Then rinse the almonds with clean water.

3. Put the almonds in the mixer. Add 2 cups of still water. Set the mixer and let it work for 1-2 minutes or until a well-mixed compound is obtained.

4. Filter the mixture obtained through a filter bag for vegetable milk. Place the bag on a container, pour the almond mixture into the bag and squeeze with your hands to filter the liquid.

5. Set the almond milk into a glass container with a hermetic lid and refrigerate for 3 days.

6. Shake the container before use since the liquid separates.

Nutrition:

Calories: 13

Fat: 9

Fiber: 12

Carbs: 21

Protein: 8

6. Eggs Benedict With Hollandaise Sauce

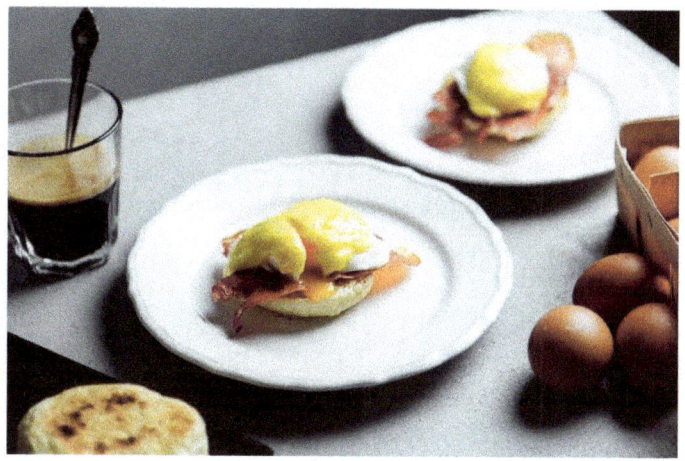

Preparation time: 15 minutes

Cooking time: 20 minutes

Servings: 2

Ingredients:

- 2 potato toasts

- 2 eggs

- 2 bacon slices

- Apple vinegar

- Salt

- Green onion

- Coconut oil

- 1 cup of water

- 2 yolks

- 1 Tbsp. of lemon juice

- Salt

- Pepper

- 1/2 cup of ghee

Directions:

1. Mix the yolks, the water and the lemon juice together in a bowl. Set the bowl in a pan filled with some boiling water.

2. Place the pan on the heat and beat the yolks until you obtain a thick and frothy compound. Add salt pepper and the ghee and keep on beating for about 5 minutes.

3. Cook the bacon and prepare the poached eggs.

4. Serve the dish placing the potato toast with one bacon slice and the egg on top of it. Add 2 spoons of sauce.

Nutrition:

Calories: 23

Fat: 11

Fiber: 12

Carbs: 25

Protein: 9

7. Shitake Mushrooms And Seaweed Omelets

Preparation time: 10 minutes

Cooking time: 15 minutes

Servings: 2

Ingredients:

- 3 Eggs

- 1/2 Cup Of Shitake Mushrooms

- 1 Tsp. 0f Seaweed Flakes

- Salt

- 1 Tbsp. Of Coconut OIL

Directions:

1. Rinse the mushrooms and cut them into pieces.

2. Beat the eggs in a bowl with seaweed flakes and salt.

3. Warmth the coconut oil in a pan and add the mushrooms, cook for 5 minutes. Season with some salt.

4. Pour the eggs in the pan and cook for 10 minutes.

Nutrition:

Calories: 21

Fat: 4

Fiber: 2

Carbs: 15

Protein: 5

8. Crunchy Green Bananas Sticks

Preparation time: 5 minutes

Cooking time: 10 minutes

Servings: 2

Ingredients:

- 2 Green bananas

- 3 Tbsp. of nuts

- 3 Tbsp. of almonds

- 1 Tbsp. of coconut sugar

- 1/2 tsp. of cinnamon

- 2 Tbsp. of coconut oil

Directions:

1. Mix the nuts and the almonds in a mixer. In a bowl, mix the compound together with the coconut sugar and cinnamon.

2. Peel and cut the bananas into strips.

3. Dip the strips into the nuts and almonds mixture.

4. Preheat a pan over medium heat with some coconut oil; cook 3-4 strips by time until golden.

Nutrition:

Calories: 13

Fat: 8

Fiber: 12

Carbs: 21

Protein: 5

9. Chinese Steamed Eggs

Preparation time: 5 minutes

Cooking time: 15 minutes

Servings: 2

Ingredients:

- 2 eggs

- 1 cup of water

- Salt

- 1 Tbsp. of minced green onion

- 1 tsp. of sesame seeds

Directions:

1. Beat the eggs with a fork, add water and salt.

2. Filter the compound into two heat resistant bowls.

3. Boil some water into a pan, when the water starts boiling put the bowl into a bamboo basket and place the basket on the pan.

4. Cover the bowls with some baking paper and the lid. Cook for 15 minutes

5. Roast the sesame seeds in a pan.

6. Season the eggs with the seeds and some minced green onion.

Nutrition:

Calories: 13

Fat: 8

Fiber: 12

Carbs: 21

Protein: 5

10. Matcha Mint Iced Tea

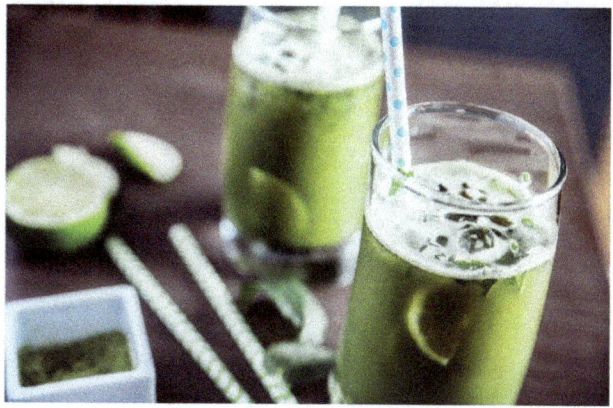

Preparation time: 5 minutes

Cooking Time: 5 minutes

Servings: 3

Ingredients:

- 4 Tbsp. of green Matcha tea ceremonial grade

- 1 lemon fresh juice

- 4 fresh mint twigs

- 4 cups of water

Directions:

1. Put the green tea in a glass, add a little bit of water and mix with milk frothier or a chosen.

2. Pour the tea in an airtight jar and add the lemon juice and the fresh mint. Add the remaining water and stir.

3. Let it rest until cold.

Nutrition:

Calories: 32

Fat: 5

Fiber: 2

Carbs: 11

Protein: 4

11. Coconut Truffles

Preparation time: 1 hour

Cooking Time: 20 minutes

Servings: 14 truffles

Ingredients:

- 1 cup of grated coconut

- 4 Tbsp. of almonds

- 4 Tbsp. of cashews

- 4 Tbsp. of walnuts

- 1 Tbsp. of honey

- 1/4 tsp. of vanilla powder

- 1 Tbsp. of coconut milk

- 3 Tbsp. of coconut oil

- 14 almonds

- Grated coconut for decoration

Directions:

1. In a mixer mix the almonds, the cashews, the walnuts and the grated coconut. (Keep 14 almonds for the filling).

2. Add the coconut oil, the honey, the vanilla powder and the coconut milk and mix again.

3. Shape 15 grams balls, and fill each of them with 1 almond.

4. Roll them into the grated coconut and refrigerate for 1 hour.

Nutrition:

Calories: 13

Fat: 15

Fiber: 6

Carbs: 15

Protein: 3

12. Soft Strawberry Cake

Preparation time: 15 minutes

Cooking time: 45 minutes

Servings: 6

Ingredients:

- 1 cup of almonds flour

- 1/3 cup of arrowroot

- 4 eggs

- 1/2 lb. of strawberries

- 3 Tbsp. of honey

- 1/4 tsp. of vanilla powder

- 1 tsp. of baking soda

- Salt

- 5 Tbsp. of ghee

Directions:

1. Beat the eggs together with the honey, add the heated ghee.

2. In another bowl mix almond flour, vanilla powder, baking soda, arrowroot and salt.

3. Mix the two compounds together.

4. Cut the strawberries into 4 pieces.

5. Pour the compound in a baking tin covered with some baking paper, add the strawberries.

6. Cook in the oven for 45 minutes (330F).

Nutrition:

Calories: 43

Fat: 17

Fiber: 8

Carbs: 21

Protein: 7

13. Chestnuts And Walnuts Cookies

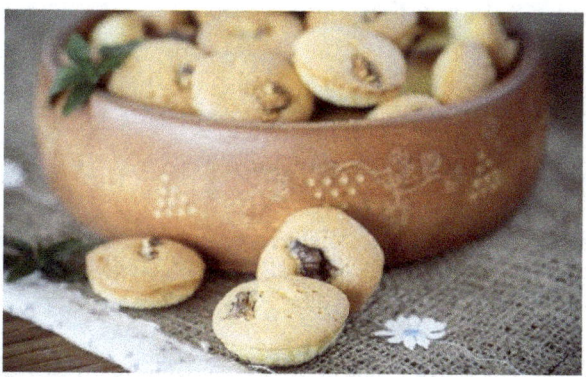

Preparation time: 10 minutes

Cooking time: 20 minutes

Servings: 13 cookies

Ingredients:

- 1 cup of chestnuts flour

- 1/2 cup of walnuts flour

- 1 egg

- 3 Tbsp. of coconut sugar

- 1/2 tsp. of baking soda

- 3 Tbsp. of ghee

- 13 walnuts (for decoration)

Directions:

1. Mix the dry ingredients in a bowl.

2. In another bowl mix the egg with the heated ghee.

3. Mix the two bowls compound together.

4. Shape 13 balls and put them in baking tin covered with baking paper.

5. Place one walnut on top of every ball and cook in the oven for 20 minutes (330F).

Nutrition:

Calories: 13

Fat: 21

Fiber: 14

Carbs: 32

Protein: 9

14. Avocado, Chocolate And Orange Mousse

Preparation time: 75 minutes

Cooking Time: 20 minutes

Servings: 3

Ingredients:

- 1 avocado

- 3 Tbsp. of cocoa powder

- 1 orange

- 1 Tbsp. of honey

Directions:

1. Cut in half the orange. Squeeze one half and cut in pieces the other one.

2. In a mixer mix the avocado pulp, cocoa powder, honey, 3 Tbsp. of orange juice.

3. Place the mixture in some cups and set in the fridge for 1 hour.

4. Decorate with the orange's pieces.

Nutrition:

Calories: 32

Fat: 5

Fiber: 2

Carbs: 11

Protein: 4

15. Spinach Crepes

Preparation time: 10 minutes

Cooking time: 10 minutes

Servings: 6 crepes

Ingredients:

- 1/4 lb. of spinach

- 3 eggs

- 2 Tbsp. of coconut flour

- 1 Tbsp. of arrowroot flour

- 1/3 cup of coconut milk

- 1/4 cup of water

- Salt

- Coconut oil

Directions:

1. Mix all the ingredients out of the coconut oil in a mixer-.

2. Grease a pan with some coconut oil; put 3 tbsp. of the compound. Cook for 1 minute then turn the crepe.

3. Repeat with the remaining mixture.

Nutrition:

Calories: 31

Fat: 12

Fiber: 7

Carbs: 21

Protein: 8

16. Pan-Fried Vegetables With Green And White Asparagus

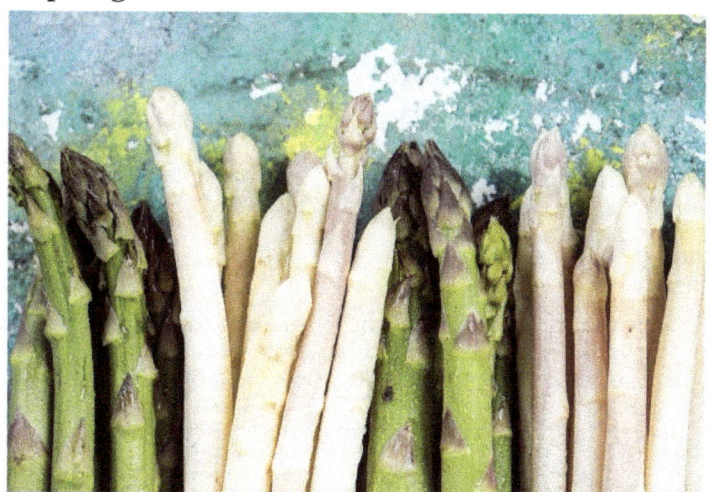

Preparation time: 10 minutes

Cooking time: 15 minutes

Servings: 4

Ingredients:

- 400 g green asparagus

- 400 g white asparagus

- 300 g tofu

- 300 g cherry tomatoes

- 1 onion

- 1 clove of garlic

- 2 tbsp. olive oil

- 4 tbsp. water

- 1 tbsp. sesame seeds

- salt and pepper

Directions:

1. Remove the skin from the white asparagus, cut off the ends, cut into small pieces and cook in boiling salted and sugar water for about five minutes. Rinse the asparagus and set aside.

2. Wash the green asparagus and cut off the ends and cut into small pieces.

3. Clean the cherry tomatoes and cut them in half. Detach the peel from the onion and the clove of garlic and dice. Cut the tofu into cubes.

4. Sear the tofu in the olive oil for about five minutes. It should get a little crispy.

5. Steam the onion in the pan. Then add the green asparagus and fry for about five minutes.

6. Mix in the garlic and fry in the pan for five minutes.

7. Add the cherry tomatoes and white asparagus and stir in. Let everything simmer with the water for about two minutes.

8. Season with a little salt and pepper to taste and garnish with the sesame seeds.

Nutrition:

Calories: 21

Fat: 9

Fiber: 2

Carbs: 21

Protein: 9

17. Spinach And Tomato Frittata

Preparation time: 10 minutes

Cooking time: 15 minutes

Servings: 6

Ingredients:

- 12 eggs

- 500 g cherry tomatoes

- 200 g spinach, frozen

- 2 onions

- 200 g ricotta

- 2 handfuls of basil

- 2 tbsp. olive oil

- salt and pepper

Directions:

1. Thaw the frozen spinach and drain the liquid.

2. Set the oven to a temperature of 200 C with a fan. Grease the baking dish with butter.

3. Whisk the eggs and mix with a whisk. Season with a little salt and pepper. Pick the basil.

4. Remove the skin from the onions, divide in the middle and cut into fine slices. Set the tomatoes and cut them in half.

5. Bring a pan with oil to temperature and fry the onions on high temperature for four minutes. Then add the tomatoes and sweat for a minute.

6. Turn the heat down and add the spinach. Steam for three minutes. Then add the basil to the pan and mix until it collapses.

7. Put the vegetables in the baking dish and spread the ricotta on top.

8. Spread the egg mixture over the vegetables and bake the frittata in the oven for about half an hour. Serve with fresh basil and tomato halves.

Nutrition:

Calories: 43

Fat: 11

Fiber: 8

Carbs: 21

Protein: 5

18. Mozzarella Omelet With Grilled Tomatoes

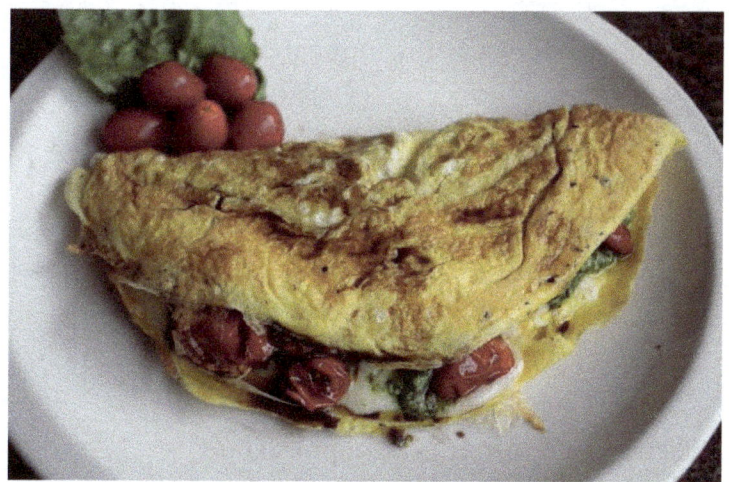

Preparation time: 10 minutes

Cooking time: 20 minutes

Servings: 2

Ingredients:

For the grilled tomatoes

- 3 medium-sized tomatoes

- 1 teaspoon olive oil

- salt and pepper

- 3 tbsp. grated parmesan

- 0.5 tsp. herbs of Provence

- Olive oil, for the baking dish

For the omelet

- 0.5 scoops of reduced-fat mozzarella, 8.5% fat

- 4 black olives

- 3 sun-dried tomatoes

- 4 eggs

- 4 tbsp. milk, 1.5% fat

- 0.25 teaspoon sweet paprika powder

- salt and pepper

- 2 teaspoons of olive oil

- 4 basil leaves

Directions:

1. For the grilled tomatoes, preheat the grill to a temperature of 200 C. Clean the tomatoes, detach the stems and cut the tomatoes in half crosswise. Brush a sufficiently large baking dish with olive oil, put the tomatoes in with the cut surface facing up, and drizzle with olive oil and season with salt. Mix the parmesan with the herbs and a little pepper and sprinkle on the tomatoes. Grill these in the oven on medium heat for about ten minutes.

2. For the omelet, dry the mozzarella. Remove the core from the olives and cut into slices. Dice the dried tomatoes and the mozzarella. Merge the eggs with the milk in a bowl and season the egg milk with the paprika powder, salt and pepper. Mix the mozzarella, olives and sun-dried tomatoes into the egg mixture.

3. Bring the oil to temperature in a non-stick pan, pour in the egg mixture and let it set over medium heat for three minutes until the underside is brown. Turn and fry on the second side as well. Halve the omelet, cover with the basil leaves and serve with the grilled tomatoes.

Nutrition:

Calories: 32

Fat: 5

Fiber: 2

Carbs: 11

Protein: 4

19. Frittata Topping With Vegetables

Preparation time: 10 minutes

Cooking time: 20 minutes

Servings: 4

Ingredients:

For the frittata

- 100 g silken tofu

- 1 tbsp. cornstarch

- 1 tbsp. soy flour

- 1 tbsp. yeast flakes

- 0.5 tsp. kala namak

- 0.5 tsp. turmeric powder

- 0.5 tsp. curry powder

- 0.5 tsp. freshly grated nutmeg

- salt and pepper

- 60 g natural soy yoghurt

For the vegetables

- 200 g zucchini

- 100 g mushrooms

- 1 small, red pepper

- 1 onion

- 1 clove of garlic

- 1 tbsp. neutral oil

- salt and pepper

Directions:

1. Drain the silken tofu for the topping. Put the soy yoghurt, the cornstarch, the soy flour and the yeast flakes in a mixing bowl and puree everything with a hand blender until creamy. Season the mixture with the turmeric, curry powder, nutmeg and kala namak, salt and pepper.

2. For the vegetables, clean, wash and dice the zucchini. Clean the mushrooms rub with kitchen paper and cut into slices. Cut the pepper in halves; remove the seeds, wash and dice. Remove the onion and garlic from the skin and chop.

3. Set the oven to 175 C. Heat the oil in a large pan and sauté the onions with the garlic until translucent. Fry the mushrooms, zucchini and bell pepper cubes over medium heat for about five minutes while stirring. Season with salt and pepper. Then take it off the stove.

4. Spread the icing on the vegetables. Bake the frittata in the stove (on the middle rack, fan oven at a temperature of 160) for half an hour until golden yellow. Let rest for 10 minutes before cutting.

Nutrition:

Calories: 25

Fat: 6

Fiber: 3

Carbs: 10

Protein: 1

20. Swiss Chard And Wild Garlic Noodles

Preparation time: 10 minutes

Cooking time: 20 minutes

Servings: 2

Ingredients:

- 150 g Greek yogurt, 10% fat content

- 1 small bunch of wild garlic

- 1 tbsp. pink pepper berries

- 1 tbsp. lemon juice

- 3 tbsp. olive oil

- Salt and sugar

- 200 g Swiss chard

- 200 g buckwheat spaghetti *

- 2 tbsp. water

Directions:

1. Remove the yogurt from the refrigerator. Clean the wild garlic and remove the coarse stalks. Finely puree the leaves with a little pink pepper, yoghurt, lemon juice and olive oil in a blender. Season the yogurt with salt and a pinch of sugar.

2. Clean the chard cut the white stems from the leaves in a wedge shape and dice. Cut the green into strips.

3. Set two liters of water to the boil in a saucepan, add two teaspoons of salt and the pasta and stir once and cook the pasta until al dente for about ten minutes.

4. While the pasta is cooking, bring the remaining oil to temperature in a pan. Add the diced chard stalks and fry for

two minutes. Attach water and steam the stems covered for two to three minutes until soft. Attach the chard leaves and cook for another two minutes. Season with salt to taste.

5. Pour the noodles into a sieve and let them drain for about half a minute, then mix with the chard and divide into two deep plates. Pour the wild garlic yoghurt over it and serve everything.

Nutrition:

Calories: 32

Fat: 5

Fiber: 2

Carbs: 11

Protein: 4

21. Chanterelle Gratin

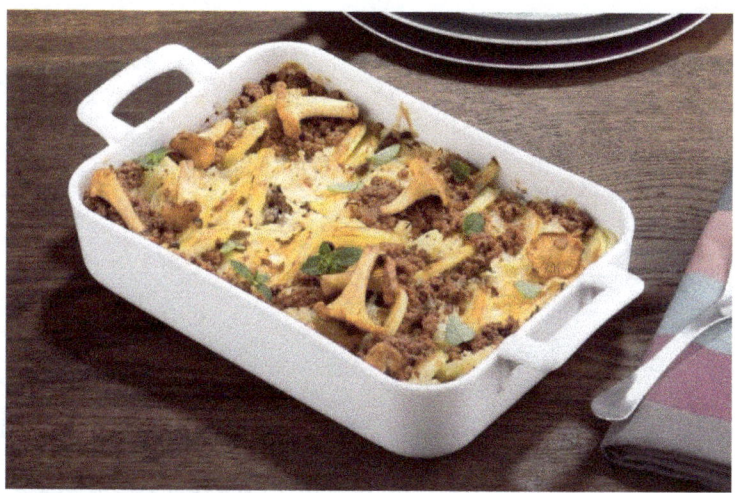

Preparation time: 10 minutes

Cooking time: 20 minutes

Servings: 4

Ingredients:

- 2 shallots

- 400 g chanterelles

- 200 g young, tender nettle leaves

- 200 g young spinach leaves

- 100 g cream

- salt and pepper

- freshly grated nutmeg

- 80 g grated parmesan cheese

- 2 cloves of garlic

- 2 tbsp. butter

- 100 ml milk

- 2 eggs

Directions:

1. Set the oven to 200 C. Remove the shell and chop the shallots and garlic. Clean the mushrooms, just rub them with a brush or with damp kitchen paper.

2. Place the nettles on the worktop (use disposable gloves), roll with the rolling pin. In this way the nettles will be broken and will not cause pain. Remove all stems. Clean and dry the nettles and spinach, then chop.

3. Dissolve a tablespoon of butter. Steam the shallots without letting them turn color. Add the garlic and let the mushrooms follow too. Sauté everything for about three to four minutes while stirring then mix in the nettles and spinach, pepper.

4. Set a casserole dish with butter and pour the contents of the pan into it. Bring the cream and milk to temperature in a saucepan, mix in the eggs, season with a little salt, pepper and nutmeg to taste. Spread the sauce over the mushroom

mixture, sprinkle with a little Parmesan and bake in the oven on the middle rack for about a quarter of an hour until the surface has a crust.

Nutrition:

Calories: 12

Fat: 5

Fiber: 1

Carbs: 4

Protein: 4

22. Pumpkin Tortilla

Preparation time: 10 minutes

Cooking time: 20 minutes

Servings: 4

Ingredients:

- 1 butternut squash (800 g)

- 2 onions

- 1 green pepper

- 0.5 frets of parsley

- 4 tbsp. olive oil

- salt and pepper

- 8 eggs

- 150 ml milk

- 100 g grated manchego

- noble sweet paprika powder

Directions:

1. Clean the pumpkin and cut lengthways in two. Scrape out the seeds and fibers. Cut the pumpkin halves into wedges and remove the skin. Cut the pumpkin flesh into one-centimeter cubes. Detach the skin from the onions and dice finely. Divide the pepper into quarters, remove the seeds and cut into strips. Wash the parsley, shake dry, pluck the leaves and chop.

2. Warmth the oven to a temperature of 180. Bring the oil to a suitable temperature in a non-stick pan (about 26 centimeters in diameter). Fry the pumpkin cubes, turning them occasionally, over medium to high heat for about three minutes. Attach the onions and peppers and cook for another five to eight minutes. Salt and pepper everything individually to taste.

3. Meanwhile mix the eggs, milk, cheese and parsley together. Season with salt, pepper and the paprika powder. Pour the

mixed milk over the vegetables and let set in the hot oven (on medium level) for about a quarter of an hour.

4. Let the omelet rest briefly. Overturn on a plate, cut into pieces. Green salad goes well with it.

Nutrition:

Calories: 13

Fat: 3

Fiber: 12

Carbs: 4

Protein: 2

23. Pumpkin And Bean Vegetables

Preparation time: 10 minutes

Cooking time: 15 minutes

Servings: 4

Ingredients:

- 500 g nutmeg squash

- 1 onion

- 2 cloves of garlic

- 1 tbsp. olive oil

- 1 tbsp. butter

- salt and pepper

- 1 teaspoon turmeric

- 1 teaspoon ground cumin

- 1 teaspoon hot paprika powder

- 150 ml vegetable stock

- 400 g green beans

- 1 tbsp. lemon juice

Directions:

1. Remove the seeds from the pumpkin, remove the skin, cut into wedges, then cut into cubes one to two centimeters in size. Skin and finely dice the onion and garlic.

2. Bring the oil and butter to temperature in a pan. Sauté the onions until translucent over medium heat. Add the garlic and pumpkin, sauté for three minutes, salt and pepper. Dust with the turmeric, cumin and paprika powder. Deglaze with the broth and simmer covered for a quarter of an hour over medium heat.

3. Meanwhile, clean the beans, cut them in half and blanch them in boiling salted water for about five to seven minutes, drain, rinse and drain.

4. Mix the beans with the pumpkin vegetables and cook for two to three minutes. Season the vegetables with lemon juice, salt and pepper.

Nutrition:

Calories: 21

Fat: 4

Fiber: 2

Carbs: 11

Protein: 4

24. Wok Vegetables With Tofu

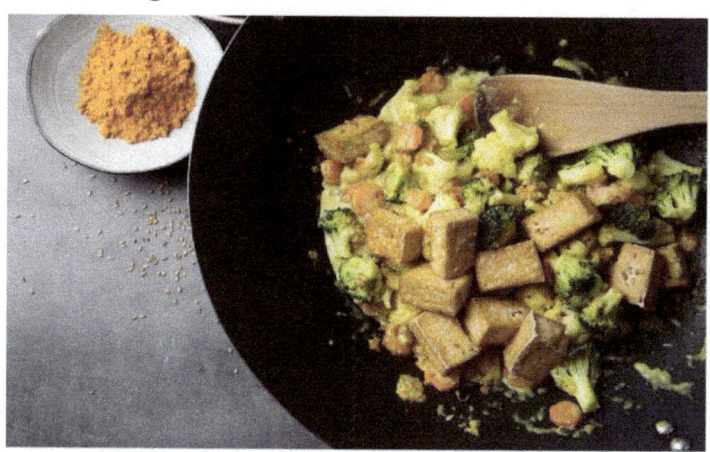

Preparation time: 10 minutes

Cooking time: 15 minutes

Servings: 4

Ingredients:

- 1 organic lemon

- 8 stalks of mint

- 3 centimeters of fresh ginger

- 1 red chili pepper

- 4 tbsp. neutral oil

- salt

- 400 g broad green beans

- 2 red peppers

- 2 spring onions

- 400 g tofu

- 150 ml vegetable stock, instant

Directions:

1. Wash and dry the lemon, rub the peel. Clean and dry the mint and remove the leaves. Remove the peel from the ginger and cut. Clean the chili pepper, remove the seeds. Finely chop the

mint, ginger and chili. Mix with the zest of the lemon, a tablespoon of oil and the salt.

2. Clean the beans and remove the end pieces, cut the beans diagonally into pieces just under one centimeter wide. Boil enough water in a saucepan, season with salt and boil the beans for about two minutes. Pour into a sieve, pour cold water over it and allow draining. Clean the peppers, cut into quarters and remove the seeds and the walls. Cut the quarters of the peppers into strips. Set and wash the spring onions and cut into rings. Drain the tofu and dice it an inch.

3. Bring the wok to temperature and add oil. Add the tofu, season with salt and fry for about four minutes until crispy. Add the vegetables and onions and stir-fry for about three minutes. Fry the herb paste, add the stock and season with salt. Serve the vegetables immediately. Rice or Asian noodles go well with it.

Nutrition:

Calories: 43

Fat: 11

Fiber: 8

Carbs: 21

Protein: 5

25. Pumpkin And Mushroom Curry

Preparation time: 10 minutes

Cooking time: 15 minutes

Servings: 2

Ingredients:

- 0.5 Hokkaido pumpkin (400 g)

- 250 g small mushrooms

- 1 onion

- 2 inches of ginger

- 2 tbsp. neutral oil

- 1 teaspoon curry paste, red or green

- 200 ml coconut milk

- 50 ml of water

- salt

- 2 teaspoons of lime juice, alternatively lemon juice

- 0.25 frets

- coriander

Directions:

1. Clean the pumpkin and scrape out the seeds and fibrous pulp. Cut the pumpkin with the skin into pieces about two centimeters in size. Clean the mushrooms, rub them with a clean cloth and, depending on the size, leave them whole or cut in half. Remove the skin from the onion and ginger and cut into cubes.

2. Bring the oil to temperature in a saucepan and fry the mushrooms over medium heat. Add the pieces of pumpkin and fry briefly. Add the onion and ginger.

3. Mix the curry paste into the vegetables and fry briefly. Pour in the coconut milk and about 60 ml of water. Season the dish with salt and the juice of the lime and cook covered.

4. Meanwhile, clean and dry the coriander, remove the leaves and chop up. Flavor the curry with salt and sprinkle with the coriander.

Nutrition:

Calories: 15

Fat: 5

Fiber: 13

Carbs: 23

Protein: 3

26. Herbal Frittata With Peppers And Feta

Preparation time: 10 minutes

Cooking time: 15 minutes

Servings: 4

Ingredients:

- 5 eggs

- sea-salt

- 1 bunch of parsley

- 4 tbsp. freshly grated parmesan

- 2 red peppers

- 1 yellow pepper

- 150 g feta

- 3 tbsp. olive oil

- salt and pepper

Directions:

1. Mix the eggs in a bowl with a pinch of sea salt. Clean and dry the parsley, peel off the leaves and chop. Stir the parsley and parmesan into the eggs. Divide the peppers lengthways, clean, wash and cut into strips. Crumble the feta.

2. Bring the olive oil to temperature in a pan. Add the paprika strips and steam for about two minutes, season with a little salt and pepper. Stream the egg mixture over it and spread the feta on top. Cover and let the frittata stand for six to eight minutes over a moderate heat. Slide on a platter, cut into pieces and serve warm or cold.

Nutrition:

Calories: 32

Fat: 5

Fiber: 2

Carbs: 11

Protein: 4

27. Vegetable Coconut Curry

Preparation time: 10 minutes

Cooking time: 20 minutes

Servings: 4

Ingredients:

- 300 g pointed cabbage

- 300 g Swiss chard

- 300 g broccoli

- 2 spring onions

- 4 centimeters of fresh ginger

- 4 stalks of basil

- 1 organic lime

- 2 tbsp. neutral oil

- salt

- 1 teaspoon of red or green curry paste

- 400 g coconut milk, pack or can

Directions:

1. Clean the vegetable parts. Cut the strong ribs flatter in the middle of the pointed cabbage. Cut the cabbage and the chard into strips one centimeter wide. Divide the broccoli, peel the stem and cut into slices about five millimeters thick.

2. Set and wash the spring onions and cut into rings. Remove the peel from the ginger and cut it first into slices, then into fine strips. Clean and dry the basil, peel off the leaves and chop. Wash the lime with hot water and dry, rub the peel and squeeze out the juice.

3. Set the oil to temperature in a large pan. Pour in the vegetables, add a little salt and fry over high to medium heat

for three to four minutes until al dente. Attach the spring onions and ginger and fry. Stir in the curry paste. Pour in the coconut milk and bring to the boil once.

4. Season the curry with the peel of the lime, two to three tablespoons of lime juice and a little salt. Sprinkle with the basil and serve. It is best to serve fragrant rice and a cucumber salad.

Nutrition:

Calories: 12

Fat: 11

Fiber: 9

Carbs: 25

Protein: 4

28. Wok Ratatouille

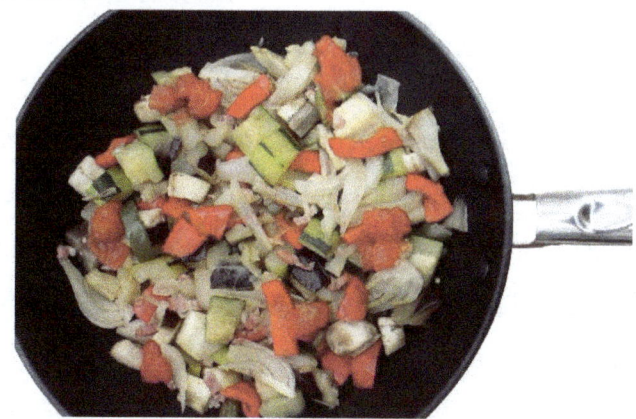

Preparation time: 10 minutes

Cooking time: 15 minutes

Servings: 2

Ingredients:

- 1 zucchini (200 g)

- 0.5 small eggplants (150 g)

- 1 red pepper

- 100 g cherry tomatoes

- 4 sprigs of thyme

- 1 sprig of rosemary

- 2 cloves of garlic

- 3 tbsp. olive oil

- salt and pepper

Directions:

1. Clean and trim the vegetables. Cut the zucchini, aborigine and bell pepper separately into half a centimeter cubes. Cut the tomatoes in half. Clean and dry the herbs and remove the needles and leaves and chop. Remove the garlic from the skin and cut into cubes.

2. Bring the wok to temperature and add two tablespoons of oil. Fry the eggplant cubes over high heat for two to three minutes while stirring. Add the zucchini and bell pepper with the remaining oil and herbs and stir-fry all ingredients for another two to three minutes.

3. Mix in the tomatoes and garlic and fry briefly. Season the dish with salt and pepper and serve immediately. Fresh baguette is served with it.

Nutrition:

Calories: 13

Fat: 21

Fiber: 14

Carbs: 32

Protein: 9

29. Tofu With Curry Mushrooms

Preparation time: 10 minutes

Cooking time: 20 minutes

Servings: 4

Ingredients:

- 500 g mushrooms, or Egerlinge

- 2 spring onions

- 2 cloves of garlic

- 0.5 frets of parsley

- 0.5 organic lemon

- 2 teaspoons of coriander seeds

- 4 tbsp. neutral oil

- 2 teaspoons of hot curry powder

- 200 ml plant cream, preferably almond or oat cream

- salt and pepper

- 500 g tofu

Directions:

1. Rub the mushrooms with kitchen paper and remove the ends of the stems. Cut the mushrooms into slices. Clean and clean the spring onions and cut into rings.

2. Remove the garlic from the skin and cut into thin slices. Clean, dry and finely chop the parsley. Wash and dry half of the lemon with hot water, finely grate the peel, squeeze out a tablespoon of juice.

3. Heat a large saucepan. Roast the coriander in it for about a minute while stirring, then remove and finely pound in a mortar.

4. Bring two tablespoons of oil to temperature in the saucepan. In it, stir-fry the mushrooms over high heat for about four minutes until the liquid has evaporated again. Attach the onions and garlic and fry briefly. Dust the curry powder over it, also fry a little. Set in the cream and bring to the boil. Season the mushrooms with the coriander, lemon zest and lemon juice, salt and pepper to taste, then keep warm.

5. Slice the tofu into thin slices and season with salt and pepper to taste. Heat the remaining oil in a large pan. Attach the tofu slices and fry for about four minutes on each side over high heat. Mix the parsley with the mushrooms. Serve with the tofu.

Nutrition:

Calories: 21

Fat: 13

Fiber: 5

Carbs: 10

Protein: 9

DINNER

30. Broccoli Wraps

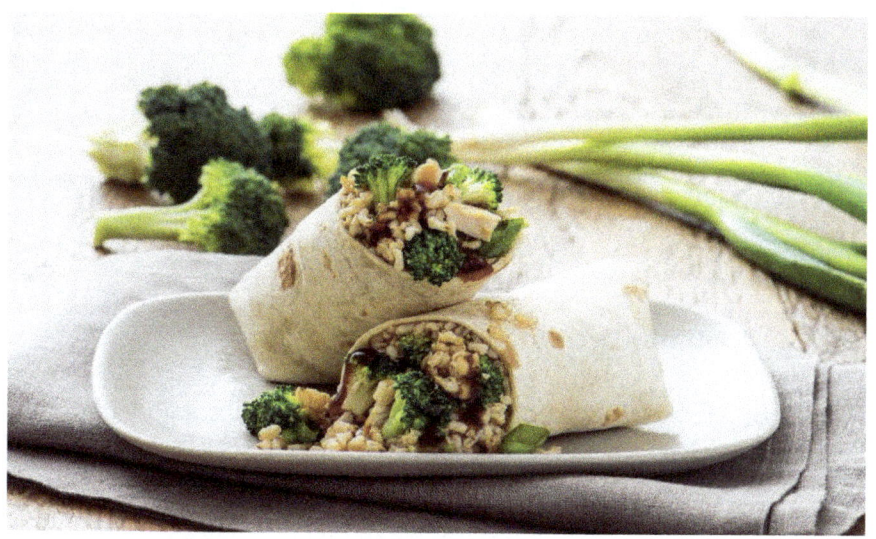

Preparation time: 15 minutes

Cooking time: 20 minutes

Servings: 4

Ingredients:

- 1 head broccoli, cut into florets

- 3 eggs

- 3 garlic cloves, finely minced

- 1 shallot, minced

- 1 teaspoon chopped fresh chives

- 1 teaspoon dried oregano

- 1 teaspoon chopped fresh parsley

- 1 teaspoon salt

- Freshly ground black pepper

Directions:

1. Preheat the oven to 350F.

2. In a food processor, press the broccoli until roughly chopped (don't over process—you want it to still be rough). Set to a microwave-safe bowl, and microwave on high for 2 minutes. Allow to cool for a few minutes, and then twist in a thin cloth or cheesecloth to remove any water (not a lot will come out, but the little that's there needs to be removed). Transfer the broccoli to a medium bowl.

3. In a small bowl, merge together the eggs, garlic, shallot, chives, oregano, and parsley, and set with salt and pepper; whisk over the broccoli, and mix until well incorporated.

4. Set a large baking sheet with parchment paper, and scoop the broccoli mixture into four equal sections. Spread each section of broccoli out until it's about 1/4 inch thick, leaving a little

room in between each. Bake and then flip and bake for another 7 minutes.

5. Detach the baking sheet from the oven, and allow the broccoli wraps to cool. Store in the refrigerator. To reheat, broil them quickly in the oven or toaster oven.

Nutrition

Calories: 143

Fat: 2.3g

Carbs: 1g

Protein: 6g

Fiber: 0g

Sugar: 0g

31. Steamed Broccoli With Hollandaise

Preparation time: 5 minutes

Cooking time: 15 minutes

Servings: 4

Ingredients:

- 1 large head broccoli

- 4 egg yolks

- 1 tablespoon freshly squeezed lemon juice

- 1/2 cup unsalted, grass-fed butter (1 full stick), melted

- 1/4 teaspoon ground cayenne pepper

- Salt

Directions:

1. Boil the broccoli. If you don't have a steamer addition for your saucepan, you can boil the broccoli for 1 to 11/2 minutes.

2. Set a saucepan of water to a simmer. To make the hollandaise sauce, in a heatproof bowl that will fit over the saucepan (without the bottom touching the water), quickly whisk the egg yolks and lemon juice together until the mixture becomes frothy and starts to expand, about 30 seconds. Set the bowl in the saucepan, and continue to whisk. Slowly drizzle the melted butter in while stirring and continuing to whisk until the sauce has doubled in size, 3 to 4 minutes.

3. Remove from the heat, stir in the cayenne and a pinch of salt, and serve immediately or keep warm over a pan of warm (not hot) water until ready to serve.

Nutrition

Calories: 240

Fat: 16g

Carbs: 2g

Protein: 19g

Fiber: 0.5g

Sugar: 0g

32. Bacon-Broccoli Bites

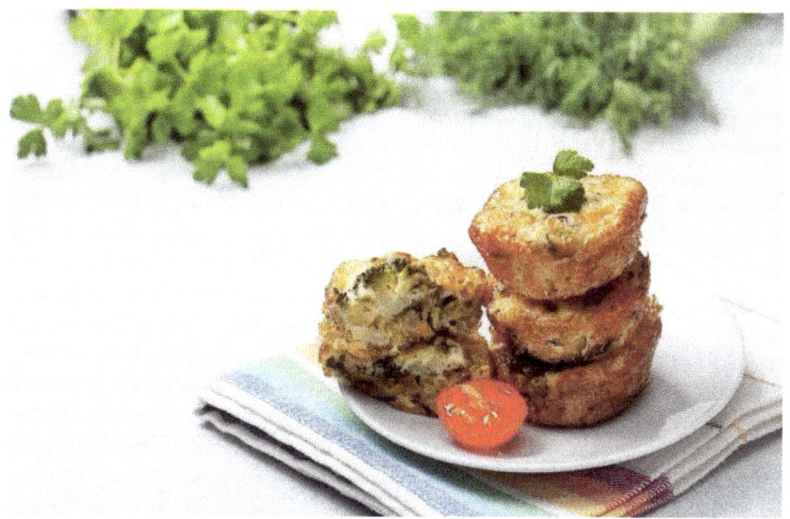

Preparation time: 15 minutes

Cooking time: 30 minutes

Servings: 4

Ingredients:

- 1 large head broccoli, cut into florets

- 1 onion, diced

- 3 garlic cloves, minced

- 3 slices bacon, cooked and chopped

- 3 eggs, whisked

- Salt

- Freshly ground black pepper

- Coconut oil, for greasing

Directions:

1. Preheat the oven to 350F.

2. Set a large saucepan with salted water to a boil. Attach the broccoli florets, and cook. Strain really well, and allow them to cool slightly.

3. In a food processor or blender, press the broccoli, onion, and garlic until pretty finely chopped. Set the mixture to a medium bowl, and stir to merge with the bacon and eggs. Season with salt and pepper.

4. Drip a mini-muffin tin with a paper towel dipped in coconut oil. Scoop the broccoli mixture into each muffin cup. If there's any leftover egg at the bottom of your bowl, pour it over the broccoli bites. Bake until set, and serve.

Nutrition

Calories: 190

Fat: 10g

Carbs: 12g

Protein: 26g

Fiber: 0.6g

Sugar: 0g

33. Broccoli-Sweet Potato Hash

Preparation time: 10 minutes

Cooking time: 20 minutes

Servings: 4

Ingredients:

- 2 tablespoons grass-fed butter or ghee

- 1/2 onion, diced

- 1 garlic clove, minced

- 2 small sweet potatoes, peeled and diced

- 1/2 pound chorizo or Italian sausage

- 1 small head broccoli, finely chopped

Directions:

1. Dissolve the butter in a saucepan. Set the onion and garlic until the onion is slightly translucent, about 5 minutes. Add the sweet potatoes, and cook for another 5 minutes.

2. Attach the chorizo, break it up with a wooden spoon, and increase the heat to medium-high. Cook and bits of it begin to get crunchy and browned, another 5 minutes.

3. Add the broccoli and stir. Cook and serve hot.

Nutrition

Calories: 138

Fat: 4g

Carbs: 1g

Protein: 23g

Fiber: 0g

Sugar: 0g

34. Pantry Basic: Homemade Nut Butter

Preparation time: 15 minutes

Cooking time: 0 minutes

Servings: 2

Ingredients:

- 2 cups raw almonds (or the nut of your choice)

- 1 to 2 tablespoons coconut oil

Directions:

1. Merge all the ingredients in a food processor until the butter reaches the consistency you like this can take up to 15 minutes. Place in a jar in the refrigerator for up to two weeks.

Nutrition

Calories: 230

Fat: 10g

Carbs: 12g

Protein: 13g

Fiber: 4g

Sugar: 0g

35. Zucchini-Noodle Salad With Lemon, Peas, And Cashews

Preparation time: 10 minutes, and 2 hours to dip

Cooking time: 0 minutes

Servings: 4

Ingredients:

- 1/4 cup uncooked cashews

- 1/2 cup water

- Salt (optional)

- Freshly ground black pepper (optional)

- 3 or 4 zucchini, spiralized or julienned into noodles

- 1/2 red bell pepper, diced

- 1/2 cup green peas

- 2 or 3 radishes, sliced

- 1/4 cup broccoli or broccoli florets

- Juice of 1 lemon

- 1/2 lemon, for garnish

Directions:

1. In a medium bowl, soak the cashews in the water for 2 hours, making sure there is enough water to cover them.

2. In a blender, merge the soaked cashews and soaking water to a creamy consistency. Season with salt and pepper (if using).

3. In a large bowl, stir well to merge the zucchini noodles, bell pepper, peas, radishes, broccoli, and lemon juice.

4. Plate the salad, drizzle with the cashew cream, garnish with lemon wedges, and serve.

Nutrition

Calories: 138

Fat: 4g

Carbs: 1g

Protein: 23g

Fiber: 0g

Sugar: 0g

36. Ratatouille

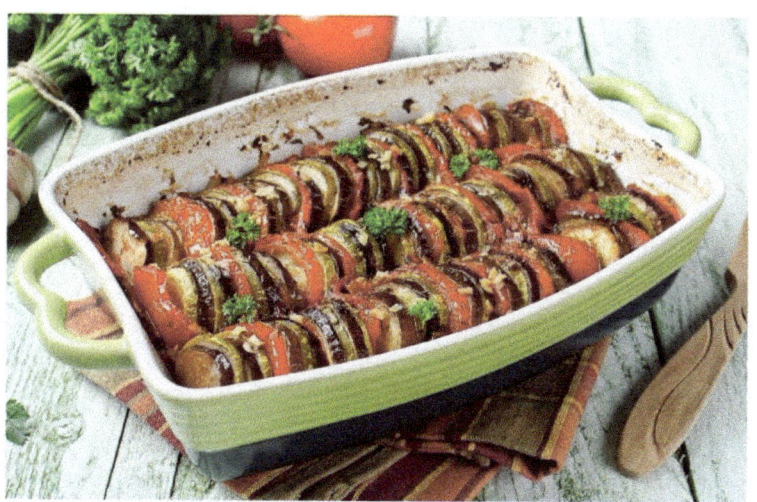

Preparation time: 15 minutes

Cooking time: 1 hour

Servings: 4

Ingredients:

- 2 tablespoons extra-virgin olive oil, divided

- 3 garlic cloves, minced

- 1 eggplant, diced

- Salt

- Freshly ground black pepper

- 2 teaspoons dried parsley

- 2 zucchini, cut into rounds

- 1 onion, cut into rings

- 1 green bell pepper, cut into strips

- 2 large tomatoes, chopped (or 10 ounces cherry tomatoes, sliced)

- 1 or 2 tablespoons chopped fresh parsley, for garnish

Directions:

1. Preheat the oven to 350F.

2. Grease a baking dish with 1 tablespoon of olive oil. In a skillet over medium heat, warmth the remaining 1 tablespoon of olive oil. Sauté the garlic until fragrant, about 2 minutes, and add the eggplant. Cook, stirring periodically, until the

eggplant begins to soften, about 10 minutes. Season with salt, pepper and the dried parsley.

3. Spread the eggplant across the bottom of a baking dish, and layer the zucchini rounds on top. Season with salt, and layer in the onion, bell pepper, and tomatoes, seasoning each layer with a pinch of salt and some pepper.

4. Bake until the vegetables are tender. Garnish with the fresh parsley and serve.

Nutrition

Calories: 321

Fat: 11 g

Carbs: 5 g

Protein: 21 g

Fiber: 3.5 g

Sugar: 1 g

37. Baked Zucchini Fries

Preparation time: 15 minutes

Cooking time: 25 minutes

Servings: 4-6

Ingredients:

- 2 large zucchini

- 1/2 cup almond flour

- 11/2 teaspoons garlic powder

- 11/2 teaspoons onion powder

- 2 eggs, whisked

- Salt

- Freshly ground black pepper

Directions:

1. Preheat the oven to 400F.

2. Chop the ends off the zucchini, and cut them in half widthwise, then lengthwise. Cut into French fry–like strips, and pat dry with a paper towel.

3. In a bowl, merge together the almond flour, garlic powder, and onion powder. Dip the zucchini fries in the egg, let any excess egg drip off, and toss them in the almond flour mixture. Season with salt and pepper.

4. Set the fries out on a baking sheet, put them in the oven, and immediately lower the heat to 350F. Cook until the fries are crisp, checking on them halfway through the cooking time and lowering the heat if they're getting brown too quickly.

5. Serve immediately.

Nutrition:

Calories: 40

Fat: 6g

Carbs: 20g

Protein: 2g

Fiber: 1g

Sugar: 1g

38. Pad Thai

Preparation time: 10 minutes

Cooking time: 20 minutes

Servings: 4

Ingredients:

- 1 pound boneless skinless chicken breast

- 2 tablespoons coconut aminos

- 2 garlic cloves, minced

- 1 teaspoon grated fresh ginger

- 1 to 2 tablespoons almond butter

- 1 tablespoon freshly squeezed lime juice, plus 4 lime wedges for garnish

- 2 teaspoons fish sauce

- 1/2 teaspoon red pepper

- 2 large zucchini, spiralized or julienned into noodles

- 1 cup bean sprouts

- 1/3 cup slivered almonds

- 2 to 3 tablespoons chopped fresh cilantro, for garnish

Directions:

1. Set a pot of water, boil or steam the chicken breasts for about 15 minutes, or until they're cooked through. Pat dry and slice into bite-size pieces.

2. In a large bowl, mix the coconut aminos, garlic, ginger, almond butter, lime juice, fish sauce, and red pepper flakes. Set aside.

3. Set a large skillet over medium-low heat, gently sauté the zucchini until they just start to become tender. Detach from the heat, and mix in with the pad thai sauce. Stir in the chicken, and serve topped with bean sprouts, almonds, cilantro, and a wedge of lime.

Nutrition

Calories: 150

Fat: 12g

Carbs: 9g

Protein: 24g

Fiber: 6g

Sugar: 0g

39. Zucchini-Spinach Fritters

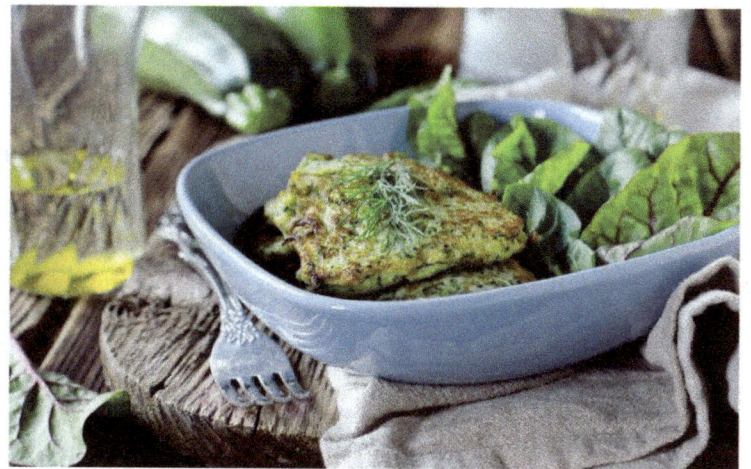

Preparation time: 5 minutes

Cooking time: 15 minutes

Servings: 4-6

Ingredients:

- 1 (14-ounce) can artichoke hearts, clear and chopped

- 12 ounces fresh spinach, washed, cooked, and drained

- 1 large zucchini, shredded

- 6 scallions, chopped

- 2 or 3 garlic cloves, minced

- 2 eggs, lightly beaten

- 1/2 cup almond flour

- 1 teaspoon salt

- 1 tablespoon extra-virgin olive oil

Directions:

1. With your hands, press as much liquid out of the artichoke hearts, spinach, and zucchini as possible.

2. In a food processor, merge the artichoke hearts, spinach, zucchini, scallions, and garlic until roughly chopped. Set the mixture to a large bowl, add the eggs and almond flour, and season with salt. Mix well.

3. Set a large nonstick sauté pan over medium-high heat, heat the olive oil. Drop heaping tablespoons of the mixture into the pan, and cook for 2 to 3 minutes on each side, flattening them a little with your spatula to make them into mini-pancake shapes.

4. Serve immediately.

Nutrition:

Calories: 21

Fat: 4

Fiber: 2

Carbs: 11

Protein: 4

40. Emergency Pasta With Zoodles

Preparation time: 5 minutes

Cooking time: 5 minutes

Servings: 4

Ingredients:

- 1/4 cup extra-virgin olive oil

- 2 or 3 garlic cloves, thinly sliced

- 1/4 hot red pepper, minced (or 1/4 teaspoon red pepper flakes)

- 3 or 4 large zucchini, spiralized or julienned into noodles

- Salt

- Freshly ground black pepper

Directions:

1. In a large sauté pan over medium-low heat, heat the olive oil. Add the garlic, and stir it around. Detach from the heat as soon as the garlic becomes fragrant—about 30 seconds—because you don't want to burn it at all. Add the hot red pepper, and pour the sauce into a serving dish.

2. In the same pan over medium heat, sauté the zucchini noodles for 3 to 4 minutes, just until slightly softened. Transfer the noodles to the serving dish, season with salt and pepper, and toss with the sauce.

3. Serve immediately.

Nutrition:

Calories: 32

Fat: 3 g

Carbs: 12 g

Protein: 1 g

Fiber: 3 g

Sugar: 1.9 g

41. Zucchini Lasagna

Preparation time: 15 minutes

Cooking time: 1 hour and 15 minutes

Servings: 6-8

Ingredients:

- 2 large zucchini

- 1 pound spicy Italian sausage

- 1 pound ground beef

- 1 onion, diced

- 1 small green bell pepper, diced

- 1 (16-ounce) can tomato sauce

- 1 cup tomato paste

- 1/4 cup red wine (optional; omit if strict Paleo)

- 2 tablespoons chopped fresh basil

- 2 tablespoons chopped fresh parsley

- 1 tablespoon chopped fresh oregano

- Salt

- Freshly ground black pepper

- 1 pound fresh mushrooms, sliced

Directions:

1. Preheat the oven to 325F.

2. With a vegetable peeler to cut the zucchini lengthwise into small, thin sheets that resemble lasagna.

3. Set a large skillet; cook the Italian sausage for 5 to 7 minutes per side, until browned. Remove from the skillet, and set aside. Attach the ground beef to the skillet, and cook for 5 minutes, using a wooden spoon to break up the beef. Attach the onion and bell pepper, and continue cooking until the beef is no longer pink, about another 5 minutes.

4. Whip in the tomato sauce, tomato paste, wine (if using), basil, parsley, and oregano, and season with salt and pepper. Once the sauce begins to boil, lessen the heat and simmer for 20 minutes, stirring frequently. Remove from the heat.

5. To assemble the lasagna, start by spreading half the meat sauce into the bottom of an 8-by-12-inch baking dish. Layer half the zucchini slices over the meat sauce. Add the Italian sausage and all the mushrooms. Continue layering the lasagna by adding the remaining meat sauce and zucchini sheets.

6. Seal with foil, and bake the lasagna for 45 minutes. Carefully remove the foil, raise the oven temperature to 375F, and bake for an additional 10 to 15 minutes.

7. Detach from the oven and allow to rest for 5 minutes before slicing. Serve warm.

Nutrition:

Calories: 21

Fat: 4 g

Carbs: 14 g

Protein: 3.1 g

Fiber: 2.7 g

Sugar: 2.9 g

42. Zucchini-Noodle Ramen

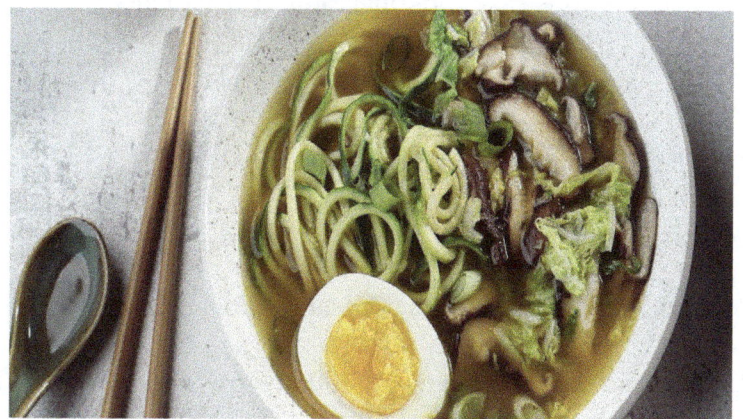

Preparation time: 15 minutes

Cooking time: 2 hours and 15 minutes

Servings: 4-6

Ingredients:

- 1 pound pork tenderloin

- 1 tablespoon salt

- 2 bunches scallions, divided

- 1 (1-inch) piece fresh ginger root, sliced

- 4 garlic cloves, crushed

- Toppings (optional): hardboiled eggs, kimchi, jalapeño peppers, fresh cilantro

- 5 tablespoons coconut aminos

- 2 tablespoons sake (optional; omit if strict Paleo)

- 11/2 tablespoons sesame oil

- 4 large zucchini, spiralized or julienned

Directions:

1. Season the pork with the salt, and refrigerate overnight.

2. Remove the pork from the refrigerator, and place in a large saucepan over medium-high heat. Add 11/2 bunches of scallions and the ginger and garlic to the pan with enough water to just cover the pork. Set to a boil, lower the heat, and simmer for at least 2 hours (although longer is better, if possible).

3. While the broth is cooking, prepare all your toppings (if using): Soft-boil the eggs (see here), slice the jalapeños and the remaining 1/2 bunch of scallions, and chop the cilantro.

4. Add the coconut aminos, sake (if using), and sesame oil to the broth. Continue to simmer, and add the zucchini noodles about 5 minutes before you're ready to serve.

5. Transfer the pork to a platter, slice it, and transfer it back to the saucepan. Serve the ramen with whichever toppings sound good to you.

Nutrition:

Calories: 21

Fat: 5 g

Carbs: 11 g

Protein: 1 g

Fiber: 5 g

Sugar: 0.3 g

43. Stuffed Zucchini Boats

Preparation time: 10 minutes

Cooking time: 1 hour

Servings: 4

Ingredients:

- 4 large zucchini

- 1 pound ground beef

- 2 tablespoons extra-virgin olive oil

- 1 onion, diced

- 2 garlic cloves, chopped

- Salt

- Freshly ground black pepper

- 3/4 cup green olives, roughly chopped

- 2 hardboiled eggs, chopped

Directions:

1. Preheat the oven to 350F.

2. Cut the zucchini lengthwise, and scoop the insides out with a spoon. Chop the inside parts, and add them to a medium bowl with the ground beef.

3. In a skillet over medium-high warmth, heat the olive oil. Sauté the onion and garlic until the onion is slightly translucent, about 5 minutes. Add the ground beef–zucchini mixture, and cook for about 5 minutes more, until completely browned, breaking the meat up as you cook it. Season with salt and pepper.

4. Detach the skillet from the heat, and add the olives and hardboiled eggs. Stir well.

5. Stuff the zucchini boats with the meat mixture, and place them on a baking sheet. Bake for 45 minutes, until tender, and serve.

Nutrition:

Calories: 17

Fat: 5 g

Carbs: 12 g

Protein: 1 g

Fiber: 3 g

Sugar: 1.3 g

44. Stuffed Squash

Preparation time: 10 minutes

Cooking time: 1 hour

Servings: 2

Ingredients:

- 2 round squash, such as acorn or 8-ball zucchini

- 2 tablespoons extra-virgin olive oil

- Salt

- Freshly ground black pepper

- 1/2 teaspoon onion powder

- 1/2 onion, diced

- 1 pound ground beef

- 11/2 teaspoons garlic powder

- 11/2 teaspoons dried oregano

- 1/8 teaspoon red pepper flakes

- 1 (14.5-ounce) can diced tomatoes, drained

- 1 or 2 tablespoons chopped fresh basil or oregano

Directions:

1. Preheat the oven to 350F.

2. Carefully cut the tops off the squash, scoop out the seeds, trim the bottoms if necessary so they will stand up straight, and season the insides with the olive oil, salt, pepper, and onion powder. Roast for 45 minutes.

3. While the squash are in the oven, in a large sauté pan over medium heat, sauté the onion until slightly translucent, about 5 minutes. Add the beef, and break it up with a wooden spoon. Season with the garlic powder, oregano, red pepper flakes, and some more salt and pepper.

4. Once the beef is no longer pink, 7 to 8 minutes, reduce the heat to low and add the tomatoes. Continue to simmer until the squash have finished cooking.

5. To serve, place each squash in a bowl or on a plate and spoon the beef mixture into the centers. Garnish with the basil.

Nutrition:

Calories: 213

Fat: 3 g

Carbs: 9 g

Protein: 3 g

Fiber: 2.1 g

Sugar: 3 g

SNACK

45. Cinnamon And Hemp Seed Coffee Shake

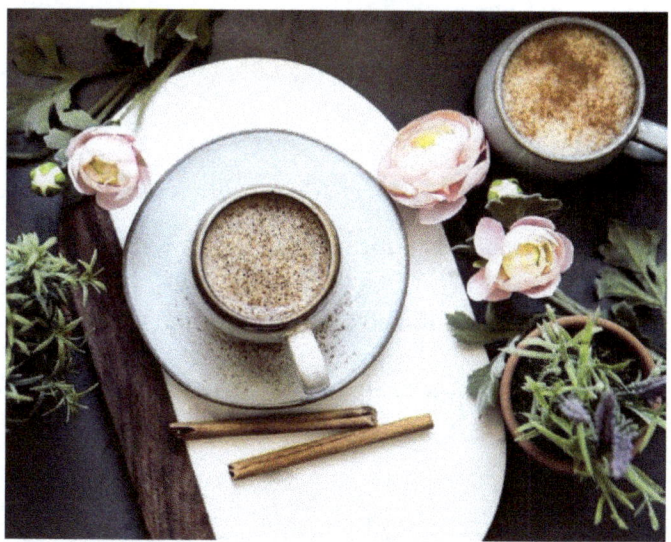

Preparation Time: 5 Minutes

Cooking Time: 0 Minutes

Servings: 1

Ingredients:

- 1 1/2 frozen bananas, sliced into coins

- 1/8 teaspoon ground cinnamon

- 2 tablespoons hemp seeds

- 1 tablespoon maple syrup

- 1/4 teaspoon vanilla extract, unsweetened

- 1 cup regular coffee, cooled

- 1/4 cup almond milk, unsweetened

- 1/2 cup of ice cubes

Directions:

1. Pour milk into a blender, add vanilla, cinnamon, and hemp seeds and then pulse until smooth.

2. Add banana, pour in the coffee, and then pulse until smooth.

3. Add ice, blend until well combined, blend in maple syrup and then serve.

Nutrition:

Calories: 410

Fat: 19.5 g

Protein: 4.9 g

Carbs: 60.8 g

Fiber: 6.8

46. Green Smoothie

Preparation Time: 5 Minutes

Cooking Time: 0 Minutes

Servings: 1

Ingredients:

- 1/2 cup strawberries, frozen

- 4 leaves of kale

- 1/4 of a medium banana

- 2 Medjool dates, pitted

- 1 tablespoon flax seed

- 1/4 cup pumpkin seeds, hulled

- 1 cup of water

Directions:

1. Set all the ingredients in the jar of a food processor or blender and then cover it with the lid.

2. Pulse until smooth and then serve.

Nutrition:

Calories: 204

Fat: 1.1 g;

Protein: 6.5 g;

Carbs: 48 g;

Fiber: 8.3 g

47. Strawberry And Banana Smoothie

Preparation Time: 5 Minutes

Cooking Time: 0 Minutes

Servings: 1

Ingredients:

- 1 cup sliced banana, frozen

- 2 tablespoons chia seeds

- 2 cups strawberries, frozen

- 2 teaspoons honey

- 1/4 teaspoon vanilla extract, unsweetened

- 6 ounces coconut yogurt

- 1 cup almond milk, unsweetened

Directions:

1. Set all the ingredients in the jar of a food processor or blender and then cover it with the lid.

2. Pulse until smooth and then serve.

Nutrition:

Calories: 114

Fat: 2.1 g;

Protein: 3.7 g;

Carbs: 22.3 g;

Fiber: 3.8 g

48. Orange Smoothie

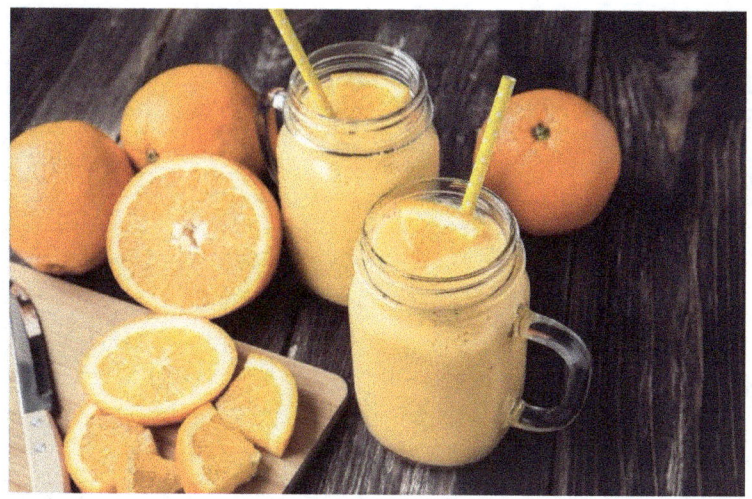

Preparation Time: 5 Minutes

Cooking Time: 0 Minutes

Servings: 1

Ingredients:

- 1 cup slices of oranges

- 1/2 teaspoon grated ginger

- 1 cup of mango pieces

- 1 cup of coconut water

- 1 cup chopped strawberries

- 1 cup crushed ice

Directions:

1. Set all the ingredients in the jar of a food processor or blender and then cover it with the lid.

2. Pulse until smooth and then serve.

Nutrition:

Calories: 198.7

Fat: 1.2 g;

Protein: 6.1 g

Carbs: 34.3 g

Fiber: 0 g

49. Pumpkin Chai Smoothie

Preparation Time: 5 Minutes

Cooking Time: 0 Minutes

Servings: 1

Ingredients:

- 1 cup cooked pumpkin

- 1/4 cup pecans

- 1 frozen banana

- 1/4 teaspoon ground cinnamon

- 1/4 teaspoon cardamom

- 1/4 teaspoon ground nutmeg

- 2 teaspoons maple syrup

- 1 cup of water, cold

- 1/2 cup of ice cubes

Directions:

1. Set pecans in a small bowl, cover with water, and then let them soak for 10 minutes.

2. Drain the pecans, add them into a blender, and then add the remaining ingredients.

3. Pulse for 1 minute until smooth, and then serve.

Nutrition:

Calories: 157.5

Fat: 3.8 g

Protein: 3 g

Carbs: 32.3 g

Fiber: 4.5 g

50. Banana Shake

Preparation Time: 5 Minutes

Cooking Time: 0 Minutes

Servings: 1

Ingredients:

- 3 medium frozen bananas

- 1 tablespoon cocoa powder, unsweetened

- 1 teaspoon shredded coconut

- 1 tablespoon maple syrup

- 1 tablespoon peanut butter

- 1 teaspoon vanilla extract, unsweetened

- 2 cups of coconut water

- 1 cup of ice cubes

Directions:

1. Add banana in a food processor, add maple syrup and vanilla, pour in water and then add ice.

2. Pulse until smooth and then pour half of the smoothie into a glass.

3. Add butter and cocoa powder into the blender, pulse until smooth, and then add to the smoothie glass.

4. Sprinkle coconut over the smoothie and then serve.

Nutrition:

Calories: 301

Fat: 9.3 g;

Protein: 6.8 g

Carbs: 49 g

Fiber: 1.9

51. Green Honeydew Smoothie

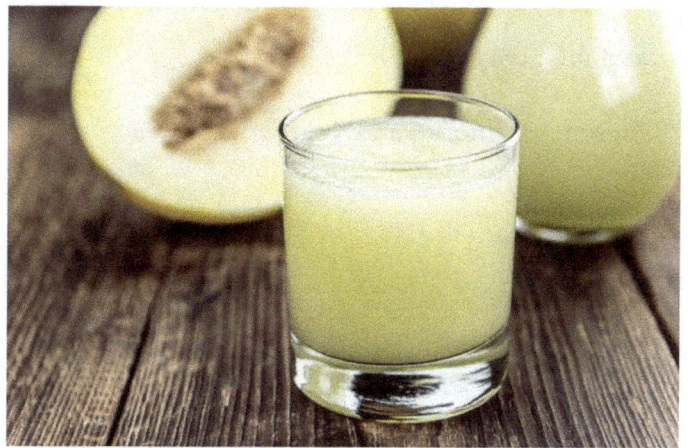

Preparation Time: 5 Minutes

Cooking Time: 15 Minutes

Servings: 4

Ingredients:

- 1 large banana

- 6 large leaves of basil

- 1/2 cup frozen pineapple

- 1 teaspoon lime juice

- 1 cup pieces of honeydew melon

- 1 teaspoon green tea Matcha powder

- 1/4 cup almond milk, unsweetened

Directions:

1. Set all the ingredients in the jar of a food processor or blender and then cover it with the lid.

2. Pulse until smooth and then serve.

Nutrition:

Calories: 223.5

Fat: 2.7 g

Protein: 20.1 g

Carbs: 32.7 g

Fiber: 5.2 g

52. Summer Salsa

Preparation Time: 5 Minutes

Cooking Time: 15 Minutes

Servings: 8

Ingredients:

- 1 cup cherry tomatoes, chopped

- 1/4 cup chopped cilantro

- 2 tablespoons chopped red onion

- 1 teaspoon minced garlic

- 1 small jalapeno, deseeded, chopped

- 1/2 of a lime, juiced

- 1/8 teaspoon salt

- 1 tablespoon olive oil

Directions:

1. Set all the ingredients in the jar of a food processor or blender except for cilantro and then cover with its lid.

2. Pulse until smooth and then pulse in cilantro until evenly mixed.

3. Tip the salsa into a bowl and then serve with vegetable sticks.

Nutrition:

Calories: 51

Fat: 0.1 g;

Protein: 1.7 g

Carbs: 11.4 g

Fiber: 3.1 g

53. Red Salsa

Preparation Time: 35 Minutes

Cooking Time: 15 Minutes

Servings: 8

Ingredients:

- 4 Roma tomatoes, halved

- 1/4 cup chopped cilantro

- 1 jalapeno pepper, deseeded, halved

- 1/2 of a medium white onion, peeled, cut into quarters

- 3 cloves of garlic, peeled

- 1/2 teaspoon salt

- 1 tablespoon brown sugar

- 1 teaspoon apple cider vinegar

Directions:

1. Switch on the oven, then set it to 425 degrees F and let it preheat.

2. Meanwhile, take a baking sheet, line it with foil, and then spread tomato, jalapeno pepper, onion, and garlic.

3. Bake the vegetables for 15 minutes until vegetables have cooked and begin to brown and then let the vegetables cool for 3 minutes.

4. Transfer the roasted vegetables into a blender, add remaining ingredients and then pulse until smooth.

5. Tip the salsa into a medium bowl and then chill it for 30 minutes before serving with vegetable sticks.

Nutrition:

Calories: 240

Fat: 0 g

Protein: 0 g

Carbs: 48 g

Fiber: 16 g

54. Pinto Bean Dip

Preparation Time: 5 Minutes

Cooking Time: 0 Minutes

Servings: 4

Ingredients:

- 15 ounces canned pinto beans

- 1 jalapeno pepper

- 2 teaspoons ground cumin

- 3 tablespoons nutritional yeast

- 1/3 cup basil salsa

Directions:

1. Merge all the ingredients in a food processor, cover with the lid, and then pulse until smooth.

2. Tip the dip in a bowl and then serve with vegetable slices.

Nutrition:

Calories: 360

Fat: 0 g

Protein: 24 g

Carbs: 72 g

Fiber: 24 g

55. Smoky Red Pepper Hummus

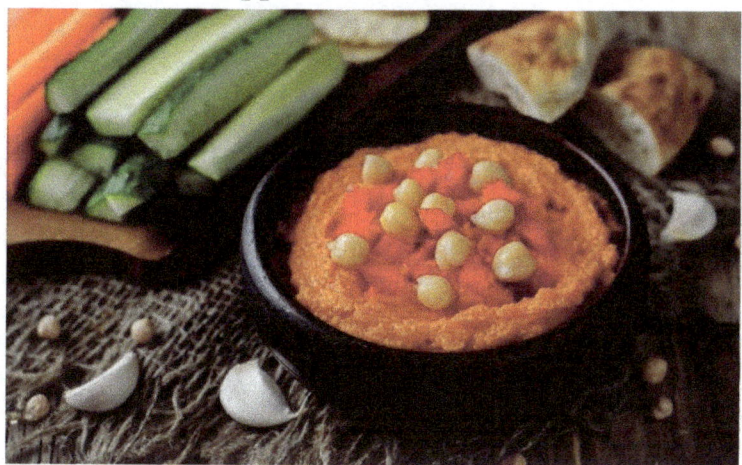

Preparation Time: 5 Minutes

Cooking Time: 0 Minutes

Servings: 4

Ingredients:

- 1/4 cup roasted red peppers

- 1 cup cooked chickpeas

- 1/8 teaspoon garlic powder

- 1/2 teaspoon salt

- 1/8 teaspoon ground black pepper

- 1/4 teaspoon ground cumin

- 1/4 teaspoon red chili powder

- 1 tablespoon Tahini

- 2 tablespoons water

Directions:

1. Set all the ingredients in the jar of the food processor and then pulse until smooth.

2. Tip the hummus in a bowl and then serve with vegetable slices.

Nutrition:

Calories: 489

Fat: 30 g

Protein: 9 g

Carbs: 15 g

Fiber: 6 g

56. Spinach Dip

Preparation Time: 20 Minutes

Cooking Time: 5 Minutes

Servings: 8

Ingredients:

- 3/4 cup cashews

- 3.5ounces soft tofu

- 6 ounces of spinach leaves

- 1 medium white onion, peeled, diced

- 2 teaspoons minced garlic

- 1/2 teaspoon salt

- 3 tablespoons olive oil

Directions:

1. Set cashews in a bowl, cover with hot water, and then let them soak for 15 minutes.

2. After 15 minutes, drain the cashews and then set aside until required.

3. Take a medium skillet pan, add oil to it and then place the pan

4. Set the onion, and cook until tender, stir in garlic and then continue cooking for 30 seconds until fragrant.

5. Scoop the onion mixture into a blender, add remaining ingredients and then pulse until smooth.

6. Tip the dip into a bowl and then serve with chips.

Nutrition:

Calories: 134.6

Fat: 8.6 g

Protein: 10 g

Carbs: 6.3 g

Fiber: 1.4 g

57. Tomatillo Salsa

Preparation Time: 5 Minutes

Cooking Time: 20 Minutes

Servings: 8

Ingredients:

- 5 medium tomatillos, chopped

- 3 cloves of garlic, peeled, chopped

- 3 Roma tomatoes, chopped

- 1 jalapeno, chopped

- 1/2 of a medium red onion, skinned, chopped

- 1 Anaheim chili

- 2 teaspoons salt

- 1 teaspoon ground cumin

- 1 lime, juiced

- 1/4 cup cilantro leaves

- 3/4 cup of water

Directions:

1. Take a medium pot, place it over medium heat, pour in water, and then add onion, tomatoes, tomatillo, jalapeno, and Anaheim chili.

2. Sauté the vegetables for 15 minutes, remove the pot from heat, add cilantro and lime juice and then stir in salt.

3. Remove pot from heat and then pulse by using an immersion blender until smooth.

4. Serve the salsa with chips.

Nutrition:

Calories: 317.4

Fat: 0 g

Protein: 16 g

Carbs: 64 g

Fiber: 16 g

58. Arugula Pesto Couscous

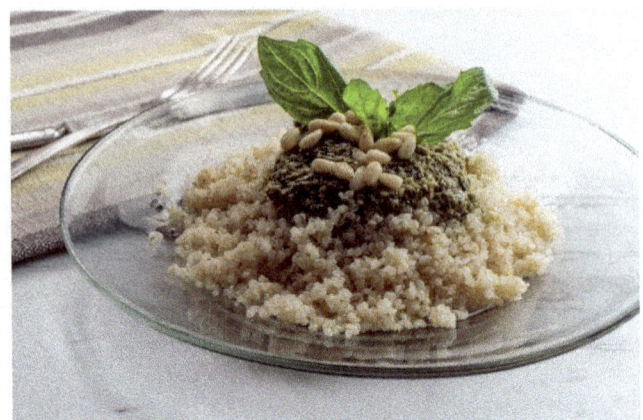

Preparation Time: 10 Minutes

Cooking Time: 20 Minutes

Servings: 4

Ingredients:

- 8 ounces Israeli couscous

- 3 large tomatoes, chopped

- 3 cups arugula leaves

- 1/2 cup parsley leaves

- 6 cloves of garlic, peeled

- 1/2 cup walnuts

- 3/4 teaspoon salt

- 1 cup and 1 tablespoon olive oil

- 2 cups vegetable broth

Directions:

1. Take a medium saucepan, place it over medium-high heat, add 1 tablespoon oil and then let it heat.

2. Add couscous, stir until mixed, and then cook for 4 minutes until fragrant and toasted.

3. Pour in the broth, stir until mixed, bring it to a boil, switch heat to medium level and then simmer for 12 minutes until the couscous has absorbed all the liquid and turn tender.

4. When done, remove the pan from heat, fluff it with a fork, and then set aside until required.

5. While couscous cooks, prepare the pesto, and for this, place walnuts in a blender, add garlic, and then pulse until nuts have broken.

6. Add arugula, parsley, and salt, pulse until well combined, and then blend in oil until smooth.

7. Transfer couscous to a salad bowl, add tomatoes and prepared pesto, and then toss until mixed.

8. Serve straight away.

Nutrition:

Calories: 73

Fat: 4 g

Protein: 2 g

Carbs: 8 g

Fiber: 2 g

59. Oatmeal And Raisin Balls

Preparation Time: 40 Minutes

Cooking Time: 0 Minutes

Servings: 4

Ingredients:

- 1 cup rolled oats

- 1/4 cup raisins

- 1/2 cup peanut butter

Directions:

1. Place oats in a large bowl, add raisins and peanut butter, and then stir until well combined.

2. Shape the mixture into twelve balls, 1 tablespoon of mixture per ball, and then arrange the balls on a sheet.

3. Set the baking sheet into the freezer for 30 minutes until firm and then serve.

Nutrition:

Calories: 135

Fat: 6 g

Protein: 8 g

Carbs: 13 g

Fiber: 4 g

60. Paleo Sweet Potato Tater Tots

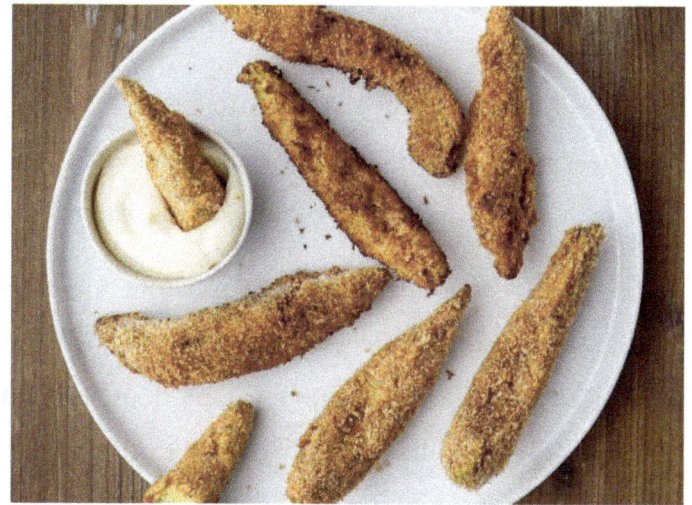

Preparation Time: 5 Minutes

Cooking Time: 20 Minutes

Servings: 4

Ingredients:

- 2 Large Sweet Potatoes (Skinned and Roughly Cubed)

- 1/4 Medium Finely Diced Onion

- 2 tablespoons of Coconut Flour

- 1 teaspoon of Garlic Powder

- 1 teaspoon of Chili Powder

- 1/2 teaspoon of Salt

- 1/4 teaspoon of Freshly Ground Pepper

- 1/2 cup of Coconut Oil (For Frying)

Directions:

1. Bring your large-sized pot of water to a boil. Add your sweet potatoes and cook for approximately 5 minutes. Drain and rinse with cold water. Shake off any excess water.

2. Place your sweet potato and onion into your food processor and pulse to break down into smaller pieces. Transfer to a large-sized bowl. Stir in your coconut flour, chili powder, garlic powder, salt, and pepper. Stir well to combine.

3. With your hands to shape the potato mixture into small cylinders. Place to the side until ready to fry.

4. Warmth your coconut oil in a heavy skillet until hot. Working in batches, add your tater tots to the skillet and fry until golden brown.

5. Serve and Enjoy!

Nutrition:

Calories: 301

Fat: 9.3 g;

Protein: 6.8 g

Carbs: 49 g

Fiber: 1.9

MEAT

61. Meatballs

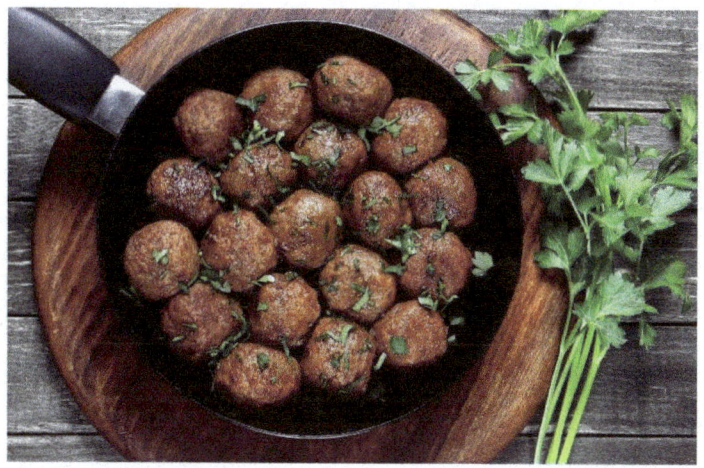

Preparation time: 10 minutes

Cooking time: 20 minutes

Servings: 4

Ingredients:

- 1 pound ground beef

- 1/2 onion, chopped

- 1/2 cup chopped fresh parsley, plus 1 tablespoon for garnish

- 3 garlic cloves, finely chopped

- 1 egg, beaten

- 1/2 teaspoon dried basil

- 1/2 teaspoon dried oregano

- 1/2 teaspoon salt

- 1/2 teaspoon freshly ground black pepper

- 1 to 2 tablespoons extra-virgin olive oil

Directions:

1. In a large bowl, merge together the beef, onion, 1/2 cup of parsley, garlic, egg, basil, oregano, salt, and pepper until thoroughly merge. Using your hands, pinch off palm-size pieces of the mixture and roll into meatballs. You'll end up with 8 to 10 meatballs.

2. Set a frying pan over medium heat, heat the olive oil. Gently add the meatballs to the pan, and brown on all surfaces, about 5 minutes per side.

3. Remove from the heat, garnish with the remaining 1 tablespoon of parsley, and serve.

Nutrition:

Calories 76

Fat 4.3

Fiber 0.3

Carbs 2.2

Protein 7.4

62. Burger Bowls

Preparation time: 10 minutes

Cooking time: 15 minutes

Servings: 4

Ingredients:

- 1 pound ground beef

- 1/2 onion, finely chopped, plus 1/2 onion, sliced, for topping

- 2 tablespoons homemade Ketchup (here)

- Salt

- Freshly ground black pepper

- 1 teaspoon extra-virgin olive oil

- 4 cups field greens or other lettuce

- Homemade Mayo (here), for topping

- Mustard, for topping

- Pickles, for topping

- Tomatoes, sliced, for topping

Directions:

1. In a large bowl, whip together the beef, finely chopped onion, and Ketchup until thoroughly combined. Season with salt and pepper. Divide the mixture four ways and form into patties with your hands.

2. Grease a large skillet or grill pan with the olive oil, and cook the burgers.

3. Divide the field greens evenly among 4 serving bowls, and place 1 burger on top of each pile of greens. Top each burger with some onion slices, Homemade Mayo or Ketchup, mustard, pickles, sliced tomatoes, or any other toppings you prefer, and serve.

Nutrition:

Calories: 301

Fat: 9.3 g;

Protein: 6.8 g

Carbs: 49 g

Fiber: 1.9

63. Taco Salad

Preparation time: 5 minutes

Cooking time: 15 minutes

Servings: 4

Ingredients:

- 1 to 2 tablespoons extra-virgin olive oil

- 1/2 onion, diced

- 1 or 2 garlic cloves, minced

- 1 pound ground beef

- 1/4 cup cherry tomatoes (optional)

- 1 tablespoon taco seasoning

- Freshly ground black pepper

- 2 to 3 cups chopped romaine lettuce, or the salad mix of your choice

- 4 to 6 tablespoons your favorite Paleo salsa, for garnish

- 1 avocado, diced or simply quartered, for garnish

- 1 lime, cut into wedges, for garnish

Directions:

1. Set a large pan over medium heat, heat the olive oil. Sauté the onion until slightly translucent, about 5 minutes. Attach the garlic, and cook for another minute.

2. Add the ground beef. Stir it around until it begins to brown, and cook all the way through, 5 to 7 minutes. If there's a lot of liquid, carefully drain it off and return the pan to the heat.

3. Add the cherry tomatoes (if using), and cook for another 2 to 3 minutes, or until they start to get wilt and some of them begin to burst. Stir in the taco seasoning, season with pepper, and remove the pan from the heat.

4. Divide the lettuce evenly among 4 bowls, and top each lettuce pile with the ground beef mixture. Garnish each salad with the salsa, avocado, and lime, and serve.

Nutrition:

Calories: 13

Fat: 9

Fiber: 12

Carbs: 21

Protein: 8

64. Hamburger And Rice-Style Ground Beef

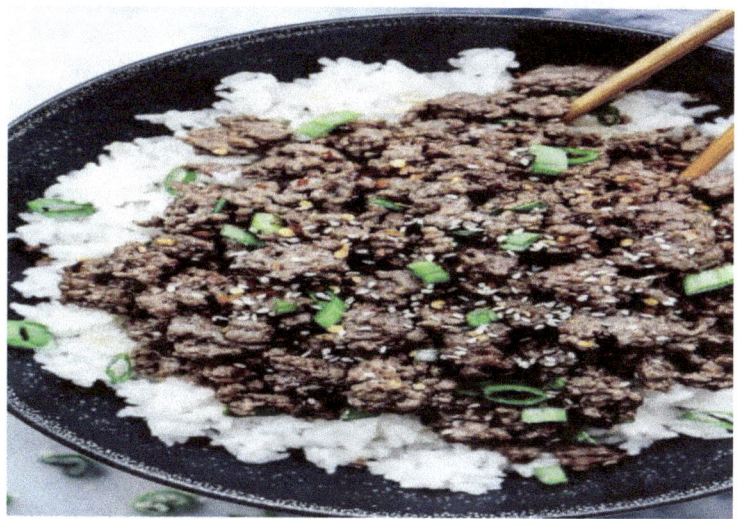

Preparation time: 10 minutes

Cooking time: 15 minutes

Servings: 4

Ingredients:

- 1 to 2 tablespoons extra-virgin olive oil

- 4 roasted red peppers, diced

- 3 carrots, diced

- 3 garlic cloves, minced

- 1 green bell pepper, diced

- 1 onion, diced

- 11/2 pounds ground beef

- 4 tablespoons tomato paste

- 1/4 teaspoon red pepper flakes

- Salt

- Freshly ground black pepper

- 1 to 2 tablespoons sliced scallion, for garnish

Directions:

1. In a large skillet over medium heat, heat the olive oil. Sauté the red peppers, carrots, garlic, bell pepper, and onion for 5 to 7 minutes.

2. When everything is slightly browned, raise the heat to medium-high and add the ground beef. Cook until browned. Attach the tomato paste and red pepper flakes, season with salt and pepper, and stir until everything is incorporated.

3. Keep warm over low heat. Scoop into bowls, and sprinkle with the scallions.

Nutrition:

Calories 32

Fat 3.5

Fiber 0

Carbs 0.1

Protein 0

65. Shepherd's Pie

Preparation time: 10 minutes

Cooking time: 45 minutes

Servings: 4

Ingredients:

For The Filling

- 1 tablespoon extra-virgin olive oil

- 1/2 onion, grated

- 1 or 2 garlic cloves, grated

- 2 celery stalks, diced

- 2 or 3 large carrots, diced

- 1 pound ground beef

- Salt

- Freshly ground black pepper

- 2 tablespoons tomato paste

- 1 teaspoon dried mustard

- 1 teaspoon dried thyme

- 1/2 fresh rosemary sprig, chopped

- 1 cup chicken broth

- 1 cup green peas (thawed if frozen)

For The Topping

- 1 large head cauliflower, cut into florets

- 2 tablespoons grass-fed butter

- 1 teaspoon garlic powder

- Salt

- Freshly ground black pepper

- 1 to 2 tablespoons coconut milk (optional)

For Assembling the Shepherd's Pie

- 1/2 tablespoon melted butter, for brushing

- 2 tablespoons sliced scallions, for garnish

Directions:

To Make the Filling

1. Set a pan over medium heat, heat the olive oil. Sauté the onion and garlic until the onion is slightly translucent, about 5

minutes. Attach the celery and carrots, and cook for 5 more minutes.

2. Add the ground beef, and season with salt and pepper. Allow to brown, about 5 minutes, and then add the tomato paste, mustard, thyme, and rosemary. Cook until any liquid in the pan begins to evaporate.

3. Add the chicken broth, cook for 5 to 7 minutes to reduce it a bit, and then add the peas. Give it a quick stir, and transfer the mixture into one baking dish or individual ramekins.

To Make the Topping

1. While the filling is cooking, fill a large saucepan with water and bring it to a boil. Attach the cauliflower to the boiling water, and cook until it is fork-tender, about 10 minutes. Rinse the cauliflower and return to the pan.

2. Add the butter and garlic powder, and season with salt and pepper. Use a mixer or immersion blender to mash the cauliflower until it is mostly smooth. If it is too thick, add some coconut milk.

To Assemble the Shepherd's Pie

1. Spread the mashed cauliflower evenly over the beef, and brush the top with the additional 1/2 tablespoon of melted butter. Set under the broiler until the mashed cauliflower becomes golden-brown.

2. Serve garnished with the scallions.

Nutrition:

Calories: 51

Fat: 0.1 g;

Protein: 1.7 g

Carbs: 11.4 g

Fiber: 3.1 g

66. Beef Tenderloin

Preparation time: 10 minutes

Cooking time: 35 minutes

Servings: 4-6

Ingredients:

- 1 (3-pound) beef tenderloin

- 3 tablespoons extra-virgin olive oil

- 3 garlic cloves, minced

- Salt

- Freshly ground black pepper

- 2 cups arugula, for serving

Directions:

1. Preheat the oven to 500F.

2. Remove the beef from the refrigerator about half an hour before you want to cook it, to bring it to room temperature. Place it in a roasting pan. In a bowl, stir the olive oil and garlic into a paste. Season with salt and pepper. Coat the tenderloin with the garlic paste, rubbing it in well with your hands. Roast for 15 minutes, or until browned.

3. Lower the heat to 375F, and cook for another 20 minutes, or until it reaches your desired level of doneness.

4. Rest the beef for 10 to 15 minutes before slicing thinly and serving on a bed of arugula.

Nutrition:

Calories 71

Fat 4.8

Fiber 0.3

Carbs 1

Protein 6

67. Classic Pot Roast

Preparation time: 10 minutes

Cooking time: 3 hours

Servings: 4-6

Ingredients:

- 1 (3- to 4-pound) boneless chuck roast

- Salt

- Freshly ground black pepper

- 2 tablespoons extra-virgin olive oil

- 1 onion, sliced

- 2 garlic cloves, minced

- 2 celery stalks, diced

- 1/2 cup red wine (optional; omit if strict Paleo)

- 1 cup beef broth

- 2 or 3 dried bay leaves

- 2 or 3 fresh thyme sprigs

- 4 carrots, chopped

- 1 cup green peas (thawed if frozen)

Directions:

1. Preheat the oven to 350F.

2. Season the roast with salt and pepper. Dip the meat for 3 to 5 minutes per side. Remove the roast from the pot, and set aside.

3. Attach the onion, garlic, and celery to the pot, and sauté until the onion is slightly translucent, about 5 minutes. Set in the wine (if using), and stir it around to deglaze the pot, scraping up any browned bits from the bottom.

4. Set the roast above of the vegetables, and add the beef broth, bay leaves, and thyme. Bring the pot into the oven, and cook.

5. Add the carrots, and cook for an additional hour. Make sure the liquid hasn't all evaporated; if it has, added a bit more.

6. Detach the pot from the oven, and add the peas. Cover the pot, and allow the peas to cook for 10 minutes while the meat rests in the dish.

7. Serve immediately.

Nutrition:

Calories 119

Fat 8.1

Fiber 1.4

Carbs 11.1

Protein 3

68. Ropa Vieja

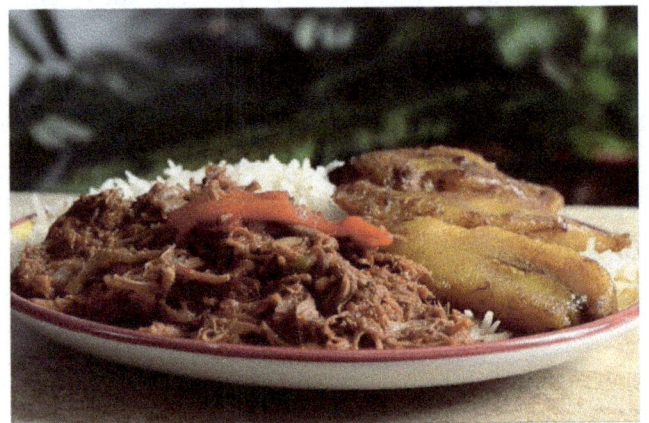

Preparation time: 10 minutes

Cooking time: 1 hour and 20 minutes

Servings: 4

Ingredients:

- 1 to 2 tablespoons extra-virgin olive oil

- 2 to 3 pounds flank steak

- 1 red onion, sliced

- 4 garlic cloves, minced

- 2 red bell peppers, cut into strips

- 2 green bell peppers, cut into strips

- 1 teaspoon dried oregano

- 1 teaspoon ground cumin

- 1/4 cup sherry vinegar

- 3 cups beef broth

- 1 tablespoon tomato paste

- 2 dried bay leaves

- Salt

- Freshly ground black pepper

- 1/2 cup chopped fresh cilantro

Directions:

1. In an oven or pot over medium-high heat, warmth the olive oil. Brown the beef (you may need to cut it in half and work in batches), about 3 minutes per side. Set aside.

2. Set the heat to medium, and attach the onion, garlic, and red and green bell peppers to the pot. Stirring frequently, cook for 5 to 7 minutes, until tender. Add the oregano and cumin, and cook for 1 minute more.

3. Attach the sherry vinegar, and deglaze the pan, stirring up any browned bits from the bottom. Cook. Add the broth and tomato paste, and stir well to combine. Set in the bay leaves, and return the beef to the pot. Season with salt and pepper. Bring the whole thing to a simmer, reduce the heat to low, and cook for another hour.

4. Set the meat to a platter, and shred it. Serve garnished with the cilantro.

Nutrition:

Calories: 32

Fat: 5

Fiber: 2

Carbs: 11

Protein: 4

69. Vaca Frita

Preparation time: 10 minutes

Cooking time: 1 hour

Servings: 4

Ingredients:

- 2 pounds flank steak

- 1 dried bay leaf

- 2 onions, 1 quartered and the other sliced

- 2 tablespoons grass-fed butter

- 2 garlic cloves, smashed

- 1/4 cup freshly squeezed lime juice,

- 3 to 4 tablespoons extra-virgin olive oil,

- Salt

- Freshly ground black pepper

Directions:

1. In a large pot, cover the flank steak (you may need to cut it in half or even quarters), bay leaf, and quartered onion with enough water to cover the meat by an inch. Set to a boil, and then simmer over low heat for 20 minutes.

2. While the beef is cooking, in a medium skillet over medium-low heat, heat the butter. Gently cook the sliced onion until it is very soft and dark brown, about 20 minutes.

3. When the beef finishes cooking, transfer it to a platter and allow it to cool before using your hands to shred it into very thin pieces.

4. Transfer the shredded beef to a large bowl, and add the garlic and lime juice. Mix well, and then allow it to marinate for 30 minutes on the counter.

5. In a large skillet over high heat, heat 1 tablespoon of olive oil. Working in batches, fry the shredded beef in a single layer until very browned and crispy, 4 to 7 minutes per batch. Flavor with salt and pepper, and remove from the heat. Repeat with the rest of the beef, adding more oil as necessary.

6. Serve each plate of vaca frita topped with some of the sautéed onions and a wedge of fresh lime.

Nutrition:

Calories 119

Fat 8.1

Fiber 1.4

Carbs 11.1

Protein 3

70. Steak Marsala

Preparation time: 10 minutes

Cooking time: 35 minutes

Servings: 4

Ingredients:

For The Sauce

- 3 tablespoons extra-virgin olive oil

- 1/2 onion, sliced

- 10 ounces mushrooms

- 2 garlic cloves, minced

- 1/2 cup Marsala wine

- 11/2 cups beef broth

- Salt

- Freshly ground black pepper

For The Steaks

- 4 large steaks (rib eyes or sirloin)

- 4 tablespoons grass-fed butter

Directions:

To Make the Sauce

1. In a medium saucepan over medium heat, warmth the olive oil. Sauté the onion until slightly translucent, about 5 minutes.

Attach the mushrooms and garlic, and cook for another 5 minutes.

2. Add the Marsala wine, and deglaze the pan, scraping up any browned bits from the bottom, and add the beef broth. Flavor with salt and pepper, and cook down until the sauce begins to thicken, 8 to 10 minutes. Set the heat to low, and simmer until ready to serve.

To Cook the Steaks

1. Preheat the oven to 400F.

2. In a ovenproof skillet over high heat, sear the steaks for 2 to 3 minutes per side, until browned. Set to the oven, and cook for 6 to 10 minutes, depending on how rare you want them. Remove from the oven, and place 1 tablespoon of butter on each steak.

3. Let rest for 10 minutes before slicing. Top with the Marsala sauce, and serve.

Nutrition:

Calories: 134.6

Fat: 8.6 g

Protein: 10 g

Carbs: 6.3 g

Fiber: 1.4 g

71. Sausage-Stuffed Dates Wrapped In Bacon

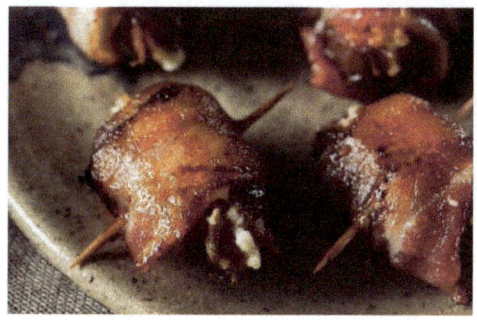

Preparation time: 15 minutes

Cooking time: 30 minutes

Servings: 8-10

Ingredients:

- 16 to 20 dates, pitted

- 1 pound spicy ground pork sausage

- 8 to 10 slices bacon, halved

Directions:

1. Preheat the oven to 400F.

2. Carefully slice each date down the middle

3. Make a roll of sausage in your hands. Stuff each date with a sausage oval. Cover each stuffed date with half a strip of bacon, and set it on a baking sheet.

4. Bake the dates until the bacon is crispy and the sausage is cooked through, and serve.

Nutrition:

Calories: 13

Fat: 9

Fiber: 12

Carbs: 21

Protein: 8

72. Candied Bacon Salad

Preparation time: 5 minutes

Cooking time: 20 minutes

Servings: 4

Ingredients:

- 10 to 12 ounces thick-cut bacon, halved or quartered

- 1/2 cup maple syrup

- 3 to 4 cups field greens (or your favorite salad mix)

- 1/2 cup pecans

- 1/4 cup Apple Cider Vinaigrette (here)

Directions:

1. Preheat the oven to 400F.

2. On a baking sheet, set out the bacon in a single layer, and brush with the maple syrup. Bake until the bacon is as crispy. Chop or crumble the bacon into bite-size pieces.

3. In a large serving bowl, merge the greens with the pecans and Apple Cider Vinaigrette. Top with the candied bacon, and serve.

Nutrition:

Calories 32

Fat 3.5

Fiber 0

Carbs 0.1

Protein 0

73. Sesame Pork Salad

Preparation time: 30 minutes

Cooking time: 10 minutes

Servings: 4

Ingredients:

-   2 tablespoons honey

- 2 tablespoons sesame oil

- 1 tablespoon coconut aminos

- 1/2 tablespoon chili oil

- 1/2 tablespoon fish sauce

- 1/2 onion, diced

- 2 garlic cloves, minced

- 1/4 tsp. freshly ground black pepper

- 1 pound pork cutlets, cut into strips

- 2 to 3 cups chopped romaine (or your favorite salad lettuce)

- 1 or 2 tablespoons sesame seeds, for garnish

Directions:

1. In a large bowl, stir to merge the honey, sesame oil, coconut aminos, chili oil, fish sauce, onion, garlic, and pepper. Attach the pork, and marinate for at least 20 minutes.

2. Warmth a cast iron pan or skillet over high heat. Add the pork, and cook until seared on all sides, about 10 minutes.

3. Put the chopped lettuce in a large serving bowl, and top it with the cooked pork. Garnish with the sesame seeds, and serve.

Nutrition:

Calories 119

Fat 8.1

Fiber 1.4

Carbs 11.1

Protein 3

74. Ground Pork Stir-Fry

Preparation time: 5 minutes

Cooking time: 20 minutes

Servings: 4

Ingredients:

- 11/2 tablespoons extra-virgin olive oil or coconut oil

- 1/2 onion, diced

- 1 green bell pepper, cut into strips

- 10 ounces mushrooms, sliced

- 1 or 2 small zucchini, diced

- 3 garlic cloves, minced

- 1 pound ground pork

- Salt

- Freshly ground black pepper

- 1/4 teaspoon red pepper flakes

Directions:

1. Set a frying pan over medium heat, warmth the olive oil. Add the onion, and sauté until slightly translucent, about 5 minutes.

2. Add the bell pepper, mushrooms, and zucchini. Allow to cool down for another 5 minutes before adding the garlic.

3. Move all the sautéed vegetables to the outside edges of the pan, and put the ground pork in the middle. Flavor with salt and pepper, and cook, stirring with a wooden spoon to break up the pieces, until the pork and the garlic begin to brown, about 5 minutes. Stir the vegetables into the center until everything is well mixed. Set the heat up to medium-high, and cook until some of the pork begins to crisp up, about 5 minutes.

4. Add the red pepper flakes, give it another stir, and serve hot.

Nutrition:

Calories: 204

Fat: 1.1 g;

Protein: 6.5 g;

Carbs: 48 g;

Fiber: 8.3 g

75. Paleo Pizza Chicken

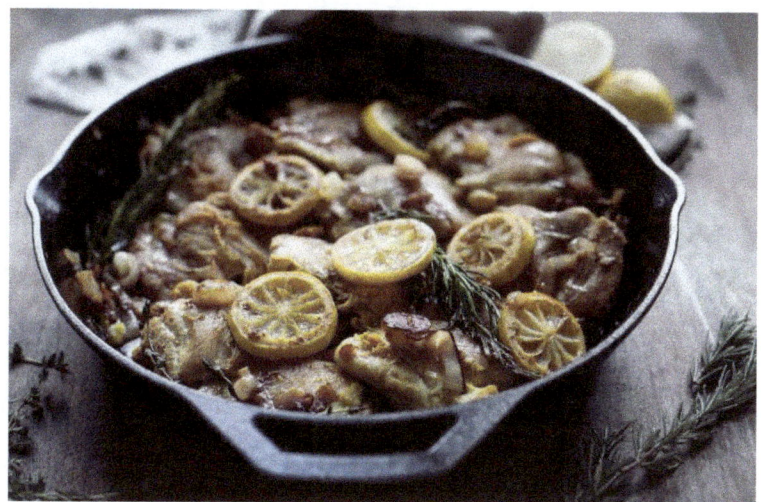

Preparation time: 10 minutes

Cooking time: 30 minutes

Servings: 4

Ingredients:

- 1 tablespoon pizza seasoning

- 2 teaspoons salt

- 1-2 tablespoon extra-virgin olive oil

- 24-30 slices uncured pepperoni

- 1/2 cup pizza sauce, sugar free

- 8 chicken thighs

Directions

1. Set the oven to around 425 degrees F and then put chicken thighs in a pan, preferably a 13x9.

2. Remove the skin from each chicken meat and then add 1 to 2 tablespoons of the sauce on the thighs.

3. Top each of the thighs with 4 to 5 slices of the pepperoni, before pulling the skin back on so that you cover the sauce and pepperoni.

4. Now drizzle the oil on the thigh and season with pizza seasoning and some salt.

5. Bake the meat until the skin is browned, or for about 40 to 50 minutes.

Nutrition:

Calories 119

Fat 8.1

Fiber 1.4

Carbs 11.1

Protein 3

76. Lebanese Lemon Chicken

Preparation time: 10 minutes

Cooking time: 30 minutes

Servings: 6-9

Ingredients:

- 2 sprigs of fresh thyme

- 2 sprigs of fresh rosemary

- 2 large shallots or 1 large onion

- 3 pounds boneless, skinless chicken thighs

- Black pepper, freshly ground

- 11/2 teaspoons flaky sea salt

- 1/2 teaspoon ground turmeric

- 2 tablespoons extra virgin olive oil

- 3 lemons

Directions

1. Obtain 2 tablespoons of lemon juice then set the juice in a large bowl along with black pepper, sea salt and turmeric.

2. Attach chicken to the bowl and toss to blend with the seasonings. Allow the thighs to marinate for a few minutes.

3. Then proceed to cut off the ends of 2 lemons before slicing them into rounds of 1/4 inch thick.

4. Next, half and peel the shallots, then discard the seeds before slicing the deseeded shallots.

5. Over medium-high heat, warm two large cast irons then add olive oil so that it coats the bottom. Divide the thighs between two pans with the skin side of the chicken facing own.

6. Cook the chicken thighs.

7. At this point, set the meat to a plate using slotted spatula or a pair of tongs. Then add in herb sprigs, shallots and the lemons to the pan.

8. Allow the ingredients to cook for 3 to 4 minutes or until the lemons are brown. Now pour half cup of water into every pan and stir as you scrap the browned bits from the pan.

9. Set the heat to medium, and then add in the meat to the pans. Cook until the flavors meld, in about 4 to 5 minutes.

10. You can now serve the lemon chicken with pan juices and shallots over cauliflower rice.

Nutrition:

Calories 169

Fat 16.1

Fiber 2.8

Carbs 4.4

Protein 4

77. Chicken With Fig And Shallot Compote

Preparation time: 10 minutes

Cooking time: 30 minutes

Servings: 4-6

Ingredients:

- 1 pint figs, finely chopped

- 3 shallots, halved and thinly sliced

- 1 lemon

- Black pepper, freshly ground

- 2 teaspoons ghee

- 1 teaspoon flaky sea salt

- 8 bone-in, skin-on chicken thighs

Directions

1. Heat the oven to 450 degrees F. Meanwhile, season all sides of the chicken with salt.

2. Heat a large skillet and then add oil or ghee to the hot pan. Set the bottom of the pan with oil then add in the chicken, with the skin side facing down.

3. Season the chicken with pepper and cook over medium-high heat until the chicken is deep golden brown, or for about 10 minutes.

4. Once done, turn off the heat, flip over the meat and then season the skin side using pepper.

5. Set the skillet to the oven and roast until the chicken is cooked through, or for around 20 to 25 minutes.

6. As the chicken roasts, zest the lemon to make thin strips before you juice it to obtain about 2 tablespoons of juice.

7. Now remove the roasted chicken from the oven and move the meat from the skillet to a plate. Cover using a foil to cool down.

8. Set off all the fat from the skillet reserving only a tablespoon. Over medium-high heat, add half of the lemon zest and the shallots to the pan.

9. Cook the mixture.

10. Set the heat to medium then add in the figs to the pan. Cook the mixture for about 2 to 3 minutes or until the figs are heated through; while stirring frequently.

11. At this point, merge in a tablespoon of lemon juice and taste the dish. Adjust the seasonings i.e. lemon juice, salt and pepper.

12. Serve the meat hot with warm compote drizzled on top. You can garnish with lemon wedges or lemon zest if you like.

Nutrition:

Calories 32

Fat 3.5

Fiber 0

Carbs 0.1

Protein 0

78. Grilled Chicken Satay

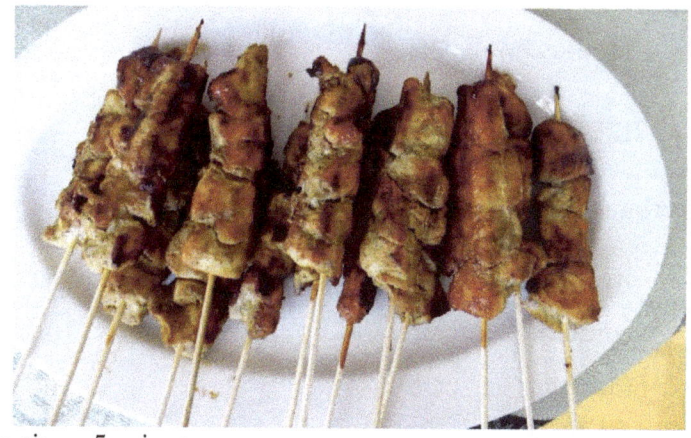

Preparation time: 5 minutes

Cooking time: 30 minutes

Servings: 2

Ingredients:

For Chicken

- Skewers

- 2 chicken breasts, boneless, skinless; 1 inch chunks

For Sauce

- 1/2 teaspoons red pepper flakes

- 2 garlic cloves chopped

- 1 teaspoons ginger, freshly ground

- 2 tablespoons coconut aminos

- 1 lime or 2 tablespoons lime juice

- 1 cup coconut milk

- 1/2 cup sunflower seed butter

Directions

1. In a food processor, set the ingredients for sauce and then combine until smooth to the consistency of a smoothie mixture.

2. Scoop about a 1/3 of the sauce to marinate the chicken chunks or the whole chicken in the fridge for about 3 hours to 48 hours.

3. Once prepared to cook the chicken, continue to preheat your grill for around 10 minutes and then turn down heat to medium i.e. 450-500 degrees F.

4. Slam the chicken using the skewers while on the grill and continue to cook for 6 minutes on each of the sides until it's done.

5. You can serve with a of cauliflower couscous garnished with pineapple or with freshly sautéed vegetables.

Nutrition:

Calories 76

Fat 4.3

Fiber 0.3

Carbs 2.2

Protein 7.4

79. Green Chile Chicken Breasts With Sauce

Preparation time: 5 minutes

Cooking time: 30 minutes

Servings: 6

Ingredients:

- 1 tablespoon sesame seeds, toasted

- 2 tablespoons whipping cream

- 1 tablespoon canola oil

- 6 chicken breast cutlets or fillets

- 3/4 teaspoon of salt, divided

- 1 clove garlic, thinly sliced

- 3 tablespoons slivered almonds, toasted

- 3 scallions, sliced, separated white and green parts

- 3/4 cup of fresh green chilies, chopped and seeded

- 1/2 cup chicken broth, reduced-sodium

- 2 cups almond milk, unsweetened

Directions

1. In a medium-sized saucepan, mix together green chilies, almond milk, garlic, scallion whites, broth and 1/4 teaspoon salt and bring the mixture to a boil.

2. Then minimize the heat and simmer for about 20-30 minutes, until the mixture is reduced by half.

3. Now set the mixture in a blender or immersion blender until smooth.

4. Using the remaining 1/2 teaspoon of salt, season the chicken and then heat some oil over medium-heat in a large non-skillet.

5. In the skillet, cook half of the chicken for about 1-2 minutes each side, until browned.

6. Then put the first batch of the chicken in the pan and then pour the sauce. Cook at low heat to simmer, for about 4-7 minutes until the chicken is tender and cooked through.

7. When done, remove from heat and then pour the sauce over your chicken.

8. Use the reserved sesame seeds and scallion greens to sprinkle on top. Serve and enjoy.

Nutrition:

Calories 169

Fat 16.1

Fiber 2.8

Carbs 4.4

Protein 4

80. Turkey Breast With Maple Mustard Glaze

Preparation time: 10 minutes

Cooking time: 30 minutes

Servings: 4-6

Ingredients:

- 1 tablespoon of ghee

- 2 tablespoons Dijon mustard

- 1/4 cup maple syrup

- 1/2 teaspoon black pepper, freshly ground

- 1 teaspoon salt

- 1/2 teaspoon smoked paprika

- 1/2 teaspoon dried sage

- 1 teaspoon dried thyme

- 5-pound whole turkey breast

- 2 teaspoons olive oil

Directions

1. To begin with, preheat your Air fryer to 350F.

2. Then brush olive oil over the turkey breast to coat it.

3. Combine pepper, salt, paprika, sage and thyme and then rub the seasonings on the turkey breast.

4. Place the seasoned turkey breast to the basket of Air fryer and cook for 25 minutes on the pre-heated oven.

5. Flip over the breast and then fry the other side for about 12 minutes. Check whether the internal temperature has reached 165F, which means the meat is fully cooked.

6. Meanwhile, mix together ghee, mustard and maple syrup in a small saucepan. After the turkey breast is cooked, turn it to an upright position and brush graze all over.

7. Then air fry for another 5 minutes until the skin is brown and crispy. Allow the turkey breast to cool when loosely covered with foil for about 5-10 minutes then slice and serve.

Nutrition:

Calories 119

Fat 8.1

Fiber 1.4

Carbs 11.1

Protein 3

81. Chicken Soup

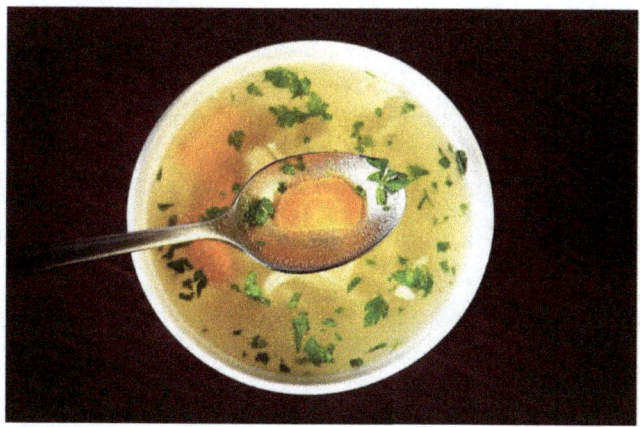

Preparation time: 10 minutes

Cooking time: 1 hour 30 minutes

Servings: 4-6

Ingredients:

- 1700ml water

- 4 chicken drum sticks

- 2 celery stalks

- 1-2 carrots

- 1 onion

- 1 tablespoon salt

- Pinch pepper

Directions:

1. Pre-heat a saucepan over medium heat, add water.

2. Wash the vegetables and dry them with paper towels.

3. Chop the ends of carrots and celery stalks. Skin the onion.

4. Put all the ingredients into the saucepan, cover with the lid and simmer for 90 minutes stirring from time to time.

5. As the soup is ready, separate the chicken meat from bones and add to the soup.

6. Pour the soup in the bowls.

Nutrition:

Calories 76

Fat 4.3

Fiber 0.3

Carbs 2.2

Protein 7.4

FISH AND SEA FOODS

82. Lemon-Butter Tilapia

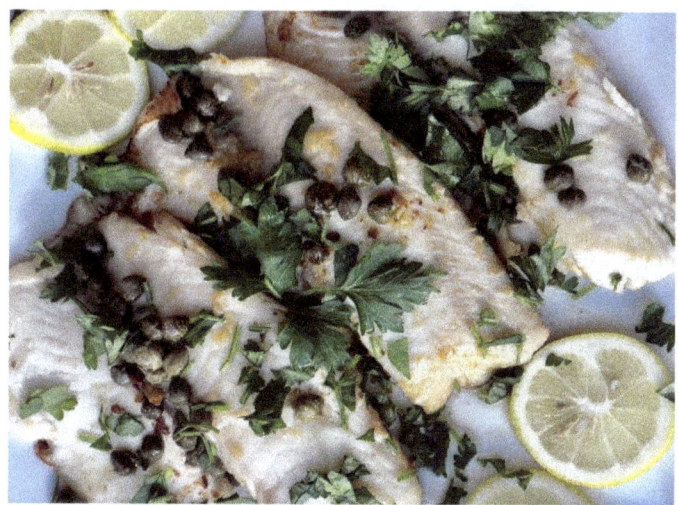

Preparation time: 5 minutes

Cooking time: 15 minutes

Servings: 2

Ingredients:

- 2 tablespoons grass-fed butter

- 1 garlic clove, sliced

- 2 (6-ounce) tilapia fillets

- Salt

- Freshly ground black pepper

- 1/2 lemon, plus 2 lemon slices for garnish

- 2 tablespoons chopped fresh parsley, for garnish

Directions:

1. In a medium pan over low heat, dissolve the butter. attach the garlic, and simmer for about 5 minutes.

2. Flavor both sides of the fish with a sprinkle of salt and pepper. Set the fillets in the pan, and cook on one side. Press the half lemon over the fish..

3. Angle the pan to gather the butter, and spoon it over the fish. Repeat a few times, and detach the pan from the heat.

4. Set the fish with a slice of lemon.

Nutrition:

Calories 32

Fat 3.5

Fiber 0

Carbs 0.1

Protein 0

83. Ceviche

Preparation time: 6 hours and 10 minutes

Cooking time: 10 minutes

Servings: 4

Ingredients:

- 1 pound halibut, diced

- Juice of 2 large lemons

- Juice of 4 limes

- 1/2 red onion, thinly sliced, divided

- 1 garlic clove, minced

- 1 jalapeño pepper, thinly sliced

- Salt

- Freshly ground black pepper

- 1 or 2 tablespoons sliced scallion, for garnish

Directions:

1. In a large glass bowl, cover the diced fish with the lemon juice and lime juice. Stir, and add half the onion. Cover and refrigerate until the fish is completely opaque. Stir halfway through the marinating time to make sure the citrus is evenly "cooking" the fish.

2. Remove the fish from the refrigerator, drain, and discard the marinade. In a clean bowl, stir to combine the fish with the remaining onion, the garlic, and the jalapeño. Season with salt and pepper.

3. Spoon into serving dishes, top with the sliced scallion, and serve.

Nutrition:

Calories 60

Fat 2.3

Fiber 0.8

Carbs 5.7

Protein 5.6

84. Sesame Marinated Fish

Preparation time: 25 minutes

Cooking time: 10 minutes

Servings: 5

Ingredients:

- 1 tablespoon sesame oil

- 1 tablespoon fresh ginger, minced

- 1 teaspoon garlic, minced

- 1 teaspoon coconut aminos

- 1 teaspoon ground fresh chili paste

- 4 white fish fillets

- Freshly ground black pepper

- 1 to 2 tablespoons sliced

- scallions, for garnish

Directions:

1. In a small bowl, stir to merge the sesame oil, ginger, garlic, coconut aminos, and chili paste. Using a brush spread the marinade onto the fish. Marinate in the refrigerator for 20 minutes.

2. Detach the fish from the marinade (discard the marinade, although you can spoon a couple of tablespoons over the fish while it's cooking, if you like). Set a large skillet over medium-high heat, cook the fish for about 5 minutes on each side, or until it turns white and begins to get flaky. Season with pepper.

3. Garnish with scallions and serve hot.

Nutrition:

Calories 169

Fat 16.1

Fiber 2.8

Carbs 4.4

Protein 4.6

85. Baked Tilapia

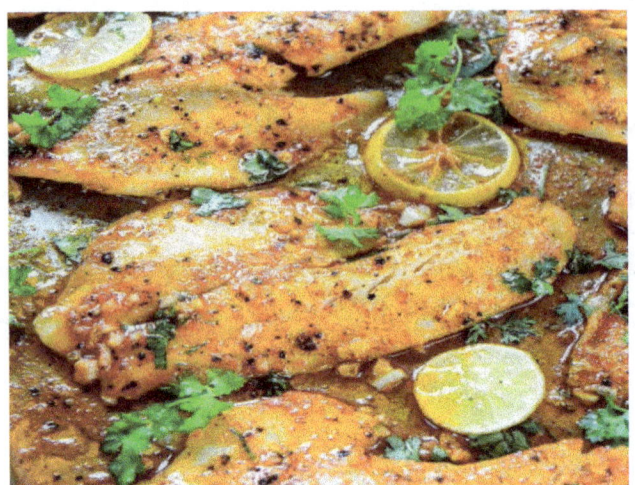

Preparation time: 5 minutes

Cooking time: 20 minutes

Servings: 4

Ingredients:

- 4 (6-ounce) pieces tilapia

- Salt

- Freshly ground black pepper

- 1/2 to 1 tablespoon garlic powder

- 1/4 teaspoon red pepper flakes

- 4 tablespoons grass-fed butter

- Juice of 1 lemon

- 1/4 cup chopped fresh parsley

Directions:

1. Preheat the oven to 400F.

2. In an 8-by-12-inch baking dish, season the pieces of fish with salt, pepper, garlic powder, and red pepper flakes. Top with 1 tablespoon of butter on each piece of fish.

3. Bake for 15 minutes, or until the fish is white and opaque throughout.

4. Detach from the oven, and pour the lemon juice over the fish. Serve with a lemon and a parsley.

Nutrition

Calories: 321

Fat: 11 g

Carbs: 5 g

Protein: 21 g

Fiber: 3.5 g

Sugar: 1 g

86. Fish Cakes

Preparation time: 15 minutes

Cooking time: 10 minutes

Servings: 4

Ingredients:

For The Fish Cakes

- 2 (6-ounce) fillets white fish

- 2 tablespoons almond flour

- 1 large shallot, minced

- 1/4 cup Homemade Mayo (here)

- Zest of 1 lemon

- Juice of 1/2 lemon

- 1/4 cup minced fresh parsley

- 2 tablespoons Dijon mustard

- 1 large egg, slightly beaten

- 1 teaspoon ground paprika

- Salt

- Freshly ground black pepper

- 2 tablespoons extra-virgin olive oil

For The Chili Sauce

- 2 tablespoons hot chili oil

- 1/4 cup apple cider vinegar

- 1/4 cup olive oil

To Serve

- 1/2 cup mizuna (or other lettuce)

- 1/2 cup arugula

- 1 carrot, julienned

- 1 small red Chile, sliced

Directions:

1. Chop the fish into a fine mince, and place in a large bowl.

2. Add the almond flour, shallot, Homemade Mayo, lemon zest and juice, parsley, mustard, egg, paprika, salt, and pepper, and mix well. Shape the mixture into four large cakes or eight smaller ones (smaller will be easier to turn over when cooking).

3. Set a large nonstick sauté pan over medium-high heat, heat the olive oil. Add the fish cakes, and allow them to brown, 4 to 5 minutes. Gently flip each one, reshaping as needed, and brown the other side, 4 to 5 minutes more.

For the chili sauce, combine all ingredients in a small bowl.

4. To serve, layer greens, carrot, and chills on serving plates, and top with fish cakes and chili sauce as desired.

Nutrition

Calories: 230

Fat: 10g

Carbs: 12g

Protein: 13g

Fiber: 4g

Sugar: 0g

87. Citrus-Baked Fish

Preparation time: 10 minutes

Cooking time: 15 minutes

Servings: 4

Ingredients:

- Ingredients: 2 lemons, sliced, divided

- 3 limes, sliced, divided

- 4 to 6 (6-ounce) fillets white fish (such as cod)

- Salt

- Freshly ground black pepper

- 1 tablespoon chopped fresh dill

- 1 tablespoon chopped fresh parsley

Directions:

1. Preheat the oven to 400F.

2. Set an 8-by-12-inch baking dish, layer half of the sliced lemons and limes to cover the bottom of the pan. Set with the fish fillets, and season with salt and pepper.

3. Layer the remaining lemon and lime slices on top, and bake for 10 to 15 minutes.

4. Remove from the oven, and serve the fish topped with the dill and parsley.

Nutrition

Calories: 170

Fat: 10g

Carbs: 2g

Protein: 22g

Fiber: 0g

Sugar: 0g

88. Poached Fish With Vegetables

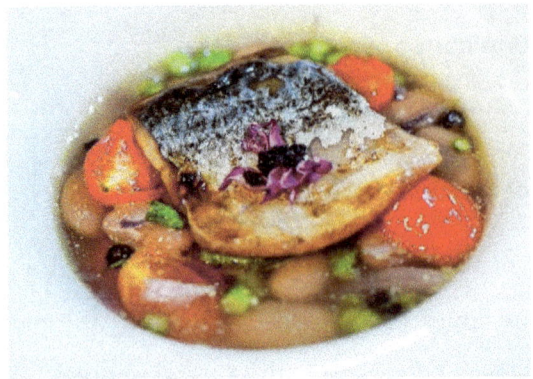

Preparation time: 10 minutes

Cooking time: 15 minutes

Servings: 2

Ingredients:

- 2 tablespoons grass-fed butter

- 2 (6-ounce) pieces white fish (such as cod or halibut)

- 1/2 cup diced onion

- 1/4 cup diced carrot

- 1/4 cup diced celery

- 2 or 3 fresh thyme sprigs, plus an extra pinch for garnish

- 1 large rosemary sprig, plus an extra pinch for garnish

- 2 or 3 fresh sage leaves (or pinch dried)

- 1 cup vegetable broth

- Salt

- Freshly ground black pepper

Directions:

1. In a skillet over medium-high heat, melt the butter. Quickly sear the fish, about 1 minute on each side. Detach it from the pan, and add the onion, carrot, celery, thyme, rosemary, and sage to the pan. Stir and sauté for 5 minutes.

2. Pour the vegetable broth into the skillet, and bring to a simmer. Return the fish to the skillet, and slowly poach until cooked throughout, 5 to 7 minutes.

3. Flavor with salt and pepper, and serve garnished with more fresh herbs.

Nutrition:

Calories: 32

Fat: 5

Fiber: 2

Carbs: 11

Protein: 4

DESSERT

89. Paleo Mayo

Preparation time: 10 minutes

Cooking time: 0 minutes

Servings: 10

Ingredients:

- 1 cup sesame oil

- 1 egg

- 1/4 teaspoon salt

- 1 tablespoon lemon juice

- 1 teaspoon mustard

Directions:

1. Crack the egg in the mason jar.

2. Add sesame oil, lemon juice, salt, and mustard.

3. With the help of the immersion blender blend the mixture until you get the smooth white sauce.

Nutrition:

Calories 201

Fat 22.3

Fiber 0.1

Carbs 0.2

Protein 0.6

90. Spicy Ketchup

Preparation time: 10 minutes

Cooking time: 15 minutes

Servings: 2

Ingredients:

- 1/2 cup tomatoes, chopped

- 1/4 teaspoon chili flakes

- 1/4 teaspoon salt

- 1/4 teaspoon raw honey

- 1 teaspoon Italian seasonings

- 1 tablespoon coconut flour

Directions:

1. Put tomatoes in the saucepan.

2. Add chili flakes, salt, and Italian seasonings.

3. Bring the tomatoes to boil and then blend them with the help of the immersion blender until you get the smooth liquid.

4. Add honey and coconut flour and whisk the mixture to get rid of lumps.

5. Simmer the ketchup for 10 minutes on the medium heat.

6. Then pour the cooked ketchup in the glass jar and let it cool.

Nutrition:

Calories 33

Fat 1.3

Fiber 1.8,

Carbs 4.8,

Protein 0.9

91. Salmon Pickle Boats

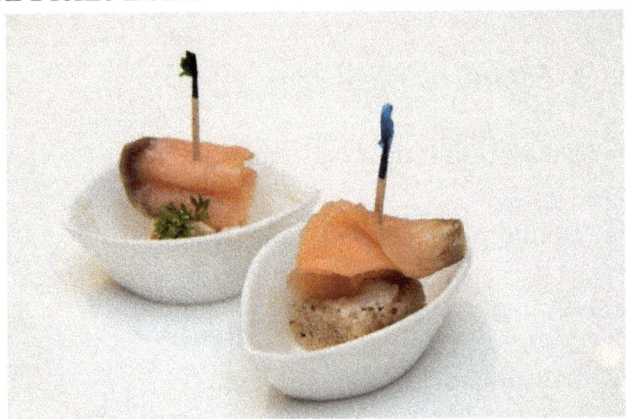

Preparation time: 15 minutes

Cooking time: 0 minutes

Servings: 6

Ingredients:

- 3 pickled cucumbers

- 1 egg, hard-boiled, peeled

- 4 oz. salmon, canned

- 1 teaspoon coconut cream

- 1/2 teaspoon minced garlic

Directions:

1. Cut the pickled cucumbers into halves.

2. Then remove the cucumber meat to get the shape of boats.

3. Mix up cucumber meat, canned salmon, coconut cream, and minced garlic in the mixing bowl.

4. Then chop the eggs and add them in the salmon mixture too.

5. Stir the mixture well.

6. Fill the pickled cucumber boats with salmon mixture.

Nutrition:

Calories 60

Fat 2.3

Fiber 0.8

Carbs 5.7

Protein 5.6

92. Sweet Potato Fries

Preparation time: 10 minutes

Cooking time: 18 minutes

Servings: 4

Ingredients:

- 2 sweet potatoes

- 1 tablespoon sunflower oil

- 1/2 teaspoon dried basil

- 1/4 teaspoon salt

Directions:

1. Skin the sweet potatoes and divide them into the French fries.

2. Then sprinkle the sweet potato fries with dried basil, salt, and sunflower oil.

3. Preheat the oven to 360F.

4. Set the baking tray with baking paper and put the sweet potato fries in it.

5. Flatten them in one layer and transfer in the oven.

6. Bake until they are light brown.

Nutrition:

Calories 32

Fat 3.5

Fiber 0

Carbs 0.1

Protein 0

93. Kale Chips With Almond Parmesan

Preparation time: 10 minutes

Cooking time: 20 minutes

Servings: 6

Ingredients:

- 1pound kale, roughly chopped

- 2 oz. nut Parmesan, grated

- 1/2 teaspoon salt

- 1 tablespoon sunflower oil

Directions:

1. Put the chopped kale in the big bowl and sprinkle with salt and sunflower oil.

2. Then add nut Parmesan and shale the kale well.

3. After this, preheat the oven to 375F.

4. Set the baking tray with baking paper and put kale inside.

5. Flatten it well and transfer in the oven.

6. Bake the chips for 20 minutes. Shake them every 3 minutes to avoid burning.

Nutrition:

Calories 113

Fat 7.1

Fiber 2.3

Carbs 9.9

Protein 4.3

94. Hard-Boiled Eggs With Chili Flakes

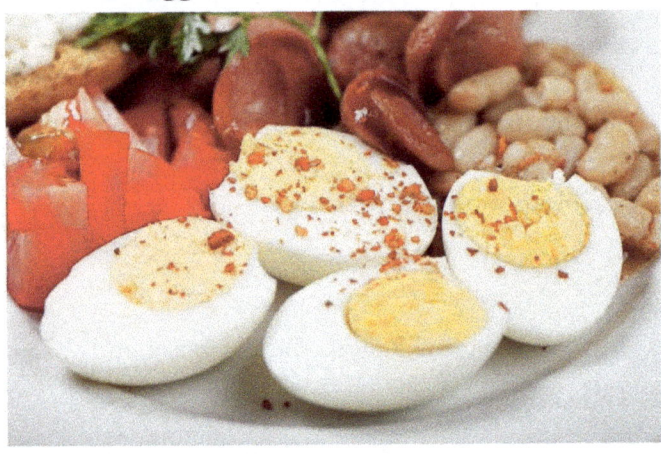

Preparation time: 10 minutes

Cooking time: 7 minutes

Servings: 2

Ingredients:

- 2 eggs

- 1 teaspoon chili flakes

- 1 teaspoon mustard

- 1 cup of water

Directions:

1. Pour water in the pan and add eggs.

2. Boil them for 7 minutes and then cool under cold water.

3. After this, peel the eggs and cut into halves.

4. Then remove the egg yolks and put them in the bowl.

5. Add mustard and chili flakes.

6. Churn the mixture until smooth.

7. After this, fill the egg whites with mustard egg yolks.

Nutrition:

Calories 71

Fat 4.8

Fiber 0.3

Carbs 1

Protein 6

95. Carrot Fries

Preparation time: 10 minutes

Cooking time: 10 minutes

Servings: 4

Ingredients:

- 2 carrots, peeled

- 1 tablespoon coconut oil

- 1 teaspoon dried dill

Directions:

1. Cut the carrots on the French fries and sprinkle with dill.

2. Then put the coconut oil in the skillet and melt it.

3. Put the carrots fries in the skillet in one layer and roast for 3 minutes from each side on the medium heat.

4. Then dry the cooked fries with the help of the paper towel.

Nutrition:

Calories 42

Fat 3.4

Fiber 0.8

Carbs 3.1

Protein 0.3

96. Roasted Nut Mix

Preparation time: 10 minutes

Cooking time: 10 minutes

Servings: 6

Ingredients:

- 3 pecans, chopped

- 1/2 cup almonds, chopped

- 1/4 cup walnuts, chopped

- 1/2 cup hazelnuts, chopped

- 1 tablespoon avocado oil

- 1 teaspoon salt

Directions:

1. Heat up the avocado oil in the skillet and add chopped pecans, almonds, walnuts, and hazelnuts.

2. Add salt and mix up the mixture.

3. Roast it for 10 minutes on the medium heat. Stir the nut mix frequently.

Nutrition:

Calories 169

Fat 16.1

Fiber 2.8

Carbs 4.4

Protein 4.6

97. Raspberry And Apple Fruit Leather

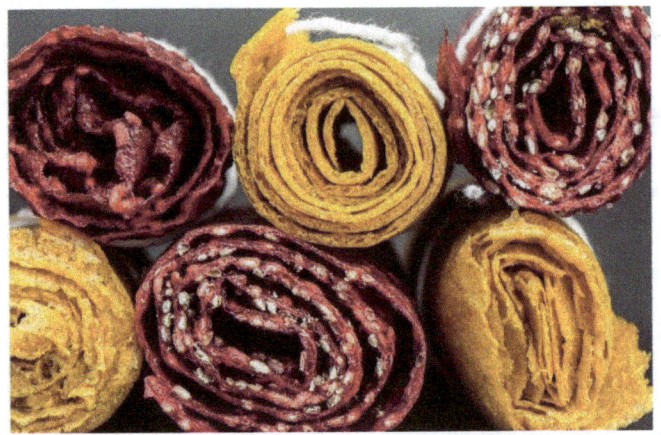

Preparation time: 10 minutes

Cooking time: 45 minutes

Servings: 6

Ingredients:

- 1 cup raspberries

- 1/2 cup apple, chopped

Directions:

1. Preheat the oven to 345F.

2. Line the baking tray with baking paper.

3. After this, put the raspberries and apples in the blender and blend until you get a smooth mixture.

4. Pour it in the baking tray and flatten well.

5. Bake the mixture for 45 minutes or until it is dry.

6. Then cut it into strips and roll into rolls.

Nutrition

Calories 20

Fat 0.2

Fiber 1.8

Carbs 5

Protein 0.3

98. Baked Apple With Hazelnuts

Preparation time: 15 minutes

Cooking time: 20 minutes

Servings: 8

Ingredients:

- 4 Granny Smith apples

- 4 teaspoons almond butter

- 2 tablespoons raw honey

- 2 oz. hazelnuts, chopped

Directions:

1. Cut the apples into halves and remove seeds.

2. Then make the medium size holes in the apple halves and fill them with almond butter, raw honey, and hazelnuts.

3. Place the apples in the tray and bake for 20 minutes at 350F.

Nutrition:

Calories 167

Fat 9

Fiber 4.2

Carbs 22.4

Protein 3.1

99. Banana Mini Muffins

Preparation time: 10 minutes

Cooking time: 10 minutes

Servings: 2

Ingredients:

- 2 eggs, beaten

- 1 banana, peeled

- 1/4 teaspoon ground cinnamon

Directions:

1. Mash the banana with the help of the fork until it is smooth.

2. Then add ground cinnamon and eggs. Stir the mixture well.

3. Pour the egg-banana mixture in the non-sticky muffin molds and bake at 365F for 10 minutes.

Nutrition:

Calories 116

Fat 4.6

Fiber 1.7

Carbs 14.1

Protein 6.2

100.   Nuts And Raisins Apple Rings

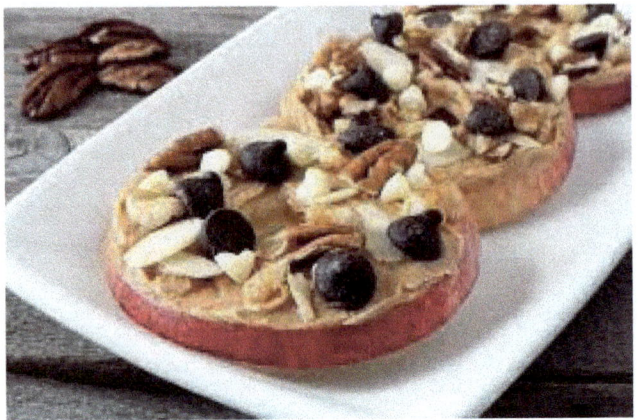

Preparation time: 15 minutes

Cooking time: 0 minutes

Servings: 5

Ingredients:

- 2 big apples

- 2 tablespoons raisins

- 2 tablespoons hazelnuts, chopped

- 1 tablespoon almond butter

Directions:

1. Core the apples and slice them.

2. Then mix up together raisins and hazelnuts.

3. Spread the apple slices with almond butter and sprinkle with hazelnut mixture.

Nutrition:

Calories 89

Fat 3.1

Fiber 2.8

Carbs 16.1

Protein 1.3

101. Chocolate Energy Balls

Preparation time: 15 minutes

Cooking time: 0 minutes

Servings: 5

Ingredients:

- 4 dates, chopped

- 3 oz. cashew, chopped

- 1 tablespoon cocoa powder

Directions:

1. Set the dates in the blender and blend until you get a smooth mixture.

2. Then add cashew and cocoa powder.

3. Blend mixture for 30 seconds more.

4. Then remove it from the blender and make 5 energy balls with the help of the fingertips.

Nutrition:

Calories 119

Fat 8.1

Fiber 1.4

Carbs 11.1

Protein 3

102.   Turkey Sticks

Preparation time: 15 minutes

Cooking time: 10 minutes

Servings: 4

Ingredients:

- 6 oz. turkey breast, skinless, boneless

- 1 teaspoon tomato paste

- 1/2 teaspoon ground turmeric

- 1 tablespoon olive oil

- 1/2 teaspoon lemon juice

Directions:

1. Cut the turkey breast on medium-size sticks (strips).

2. Then mix up together tomato paste and olive oil.

3. Add lemon juice and ground turmeric.

4. After this, mix up turkey sticks and oil mixture.

5. Preheat the skillet until it is hot.

6. Put the turkey sticks in the skillet in one layer and roast them for 5 minutes from each side or until they turkey sticks are a little bit crunchy.

Nutrition:

Calories 76

Fat 4.3

Fiber 0.3

Carbs 2.2

Protein 7.4

103.   Veggie Sticks

Preparation time: 10 minutes

Cooking time: 0 minutes

Servings: 4

Ingredients:

- 1 red sweet pepper

- 2 celery stalks

- 1 carrot, peeled

- 1 teaspoon coconut cream

- 1/4 teaspoon tahini paste

Directions:

1. Cut the sweet pepper, celery stalk, and carrot into the sticks.

2. Then put them in the plate side-by-side and sprinkle with coconut cream and tahini paste.

Nutrition:

Calories 22

Fat 0.6

Fiber 1

Carbs 4.1

Protein 0.6

CONCLUSION

The Paleo diet is a lifestyle answer that has been steadily gaining popularity these days. Many people are finding this diet very beneficial to their health. It is a natural diet that focuses on whole, unprocessed foods.

With the Paleo diet, you can lose weight and feel healthier. The Paleo diet is low in sugar. It is free of grains, dairy products, legumes, refined carbohydrates, and processed foods. This means that you get to eat natural foods rich in vitamins, minerals, antioxidants, and fiber.

The Paleo diet helps in the prevention of various diseases. Some of the Paleo diet benefits include an improved immune system and a reduction of chances of developing certain kinds of cancer and heart disease. This paleo diet is a manner of eating that became popular in the early 2000s. It's a lifestyle that hunter-gatherers have practiced for millions of years before the advent of agriculture. One of the main ideas behind this is that we are evolved to eat foods that are in season at the time. It's a way to ensure we get nutrients from our food. A straightforward way to implement this way of eating is to find whole, fresh foods that are in season at the time. The paleo diet doesn't encourage consuming processed foods, fast food, or refined sugars or oils. It's considered ideal for keeping your mind and body healthy. It's also great for weight loss since it encourages eating fresh foods and minimizes your exposure to chemicals such as preservatives and artificial additives. The paleo diet is a lifestyle of Paleolithic humans.

This means that the way they ate was different from the way we eat today. This diet was designed as a way to mimic our ancestor's eating habits.

The paleo diet is a center point on eating foods that are rich in vitamins and minerals. These foods include fish, meats, vegetables, fruits, nuts, and seeds. This diet also encourages low glycemic fruits and vegetables that are low on the glycemic index.

As beneficial as this diet may be to your health, it also has drawbacks. For example- individuals following the paleo diet can suffer from nutrient deficiencies. This type of diet can also lead to a greater incidence of health issues like acne and cancer.

However you cope with these issues, you should know about what the paleo diet is and how it's used today.

Lightning Source UK Ltd.
Milton Keynes UK
UKHW021820160421
382091UK00005B/97